Evidence-based Practice for Nurses

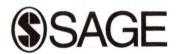

2ND Edition

Evidence-based Practice for Nurses

Janet Barker

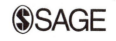

Los Angeles | London | New Delhi
Singapore | Washington DC

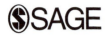

Los Angeles | London | New Delhi
Singapore | Washington DC

SAGE Publications Ltd
1 Oliver's Yard
55 City Road
London EC1Y 1SP

SAGE Publications Inc.
2455 Teller Road
Thousand Oaks, California 91320

SAGE Publications India Pvt Ltd
B 1/I 1 Mohan Cooperative Industrial Area
Mathura Road
New Delhi 110 044

SAGE Publications Asia-Pacific Pte Ltd
3 Church Street
#10-04 Samsung Hub
Singapore 049483

Editor: Alex Clabburn
Assistant editor: Emma Milman
Production editor: Katie Forsythe
Copyeditor: Jane Fricker
Proofreader: Bryan Campbell
Indexer: Caroline Eley
Marketing manager: Tamara Navaratnam
Cover design: Naomi Robinson
Typeset by: C&M Digitals (P) Ltd, Chennai, India
Printed by MPG Printgroup, UK

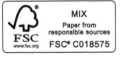

MIX
Paper from
responsible sources
FSC® C018575
www.fsc.org

Library of Congress Control Number: 2012944839

British Library Cataloguing in Publication data

A catalogue record for this book is available from
the British Library

ISBN 978-1-4462-5228-4
ISBN 978-1-4462-5229-1 (pbk)

Contents

About the Author

Dr Janet Barker has been involved in nursing for 40 years, starting as a cadet nurse at 16 years of age in an orthopaedic hospital, moving into general nursing and finally working as a mental health nurse, in both inpatient and community settings. The last 20 years have been spent in nurse education. Janet has vast experience of organising and delivering undergraduate pre-registration nursing courses, taking on the role of Course Director of the Diploma/BSc (Hons) in Nursing programme at the University of Nottingham, School of Nursing, Midwifery and Physiotherapy in 2005. Janet received the University of Nottingham 'Dearing Award' in 2011 in recognition of her 'outstanding contribution to the development of teaching and student learning'. She retired as Associate Professor at the University of Nottingham in July 2011, however continues to keep abreast of current developments in nursing.

Preface

Welcome to the second edition of *Evidence-Based Practice for Nurses*. Evidence-based practice (EBP) remains an essential component of nursing with the Nursing and Midwifery Council (NMC) (2008) identifying that registered nurses 'must deliver care based on best evidence or best practice'. The Standards for Pre-Registration Nurse Education (NMC, 2010) state that newly qualified nurses must 'be responsible and accountable for safe, person-centred, evidence-based nursing practice'. Pearson et al. (2007) identify that whatever position you hold in nursing – student or registered nurse, staff nurse or service manager – you are expected to be able to assess the quality of evidence used in practice and deliver care supported by best evidence. However, as you will see in the following chapters, there is a great deal of debate surrounding EBP and what it means in reality for nursing and the delivery/management of care.

There are various skills and knowledge bases which you need to develop if you are to meet the NMC requirements, the challenges of modern practice and to fulfil your responsibilities as an accountable practitioner. The intention here is to provide you with a resource to help you navigate the process of EBP, develop the necessary knowledge and skills and ensure your practice is based on best evidence.

There are a number of ways you can use this book. If you are new to the concept of EBP you may want to work through the chapters at your own pace and gain the necessary knowledge and skills in a step-by-step way. If you already have some insight into EBP, you may want to dip into various chapters as appropriate to your learning needs. Each chapter begins with a list of learning outcomes so you can identify what you should know at the end of it and concludes with a summary of the main points, suggestions for further reading and useful e-resources. Key terms are highlighted and definitions given in the glossary.

What's in the book?

The book falls into three parts, Part 1 looks at the critical elements of EBP – evidence, clinical expertise, patient preference, local context – and how to find evidence. Chapter 1 considers what EBP is and why it is important that nurses understand and develop the necessary knowledge and skills. Chapter 2 explores issues in relation to what knowledge is and where it comes from; what knowledge is seen as underpinning the practice of nursing; what counts as good and appropriate evidence; and how to identify what it is that you want to know. Chapter 3 addresses issues related to patient preferences and local context. Chapter 4 considers issues related to clinical judgement, expertise and decision making. Chapter 5 discusses how you go about finding the evidence and developing a search strategy.

Part 2 provides an opportunity to explore the knowledge and skills associated with the critical appraisal of evidence, beginning with Chapter 6, which identifies what is meant by critical appraisal and its role in the EBP process. Chapters 7 and 8 look at critical appraisal specifically in relation to quantitative and qualitative research respectively. Chapter 9 considers issues related to systematic review and its place in EBP. Critical appraisal tools to help with this process are provided in the appendices.

Finally, Part 3 looks at how to make changes to practice once you have found and critically appraised the evidence. Chapter 10 considers how you integrate evidence into your own practice and how you can begin to influence change generally and help develop an EBP culture in the practice setting. Chapter 11 discusses issues related to your professional development, and how you ensure your practice continues to be evidence-based through the use of reflection and portfolio work. Templates for activities are provided in the appendices.

Each section ends with a quiz to enable you to test your learning so far. At various points activities are used to help you develop your skills in certain areas. To help you consolidate your learning in relation to the issues discussed, each chapter ends with an EBP activity.

I hope you will find the book a useful resource, one that helps you to develop the knowledge and skills needed to ensure patients receive the best care possible – based on good evidence and aimed at achieving positive outcomes.

Part 1

Introducing Evidence-Based Practice

Chapter 1

Introduction: What is Evidence-Based Practice?

Learning Outcomes

By the end of the chapter you will be able to:

- define evidence-based practice;
- understand how evidence-based practice came into being;
- discuss the pros and cons of evidence-based practice;
- identify the components of evidence-based practice and the skills associated with it;
- consider why your practice needs to be evidence-based.

Introduction

Many terms are used in relation to evidence-based practice (EBP) – evidence-based nursing, evidence-based nursing practice, evidence-based medicine, evidence-based decision making and evidence-based healthcare. The idea of EBP is at the forefront of healthcare discussions, leaving Rycroft-Malone et al. to suggest that it has become a global phenomenon, with **evidence** being something of a 'buzz word' (2004a: 82), and Porter and O'Halloran (2012: 18) proposing it to be 'one of the most significant developments in health care in the last couple of decades'. A simple search of the CINAHL (Cumulative Index to Nursing and Allied Health Literature) database, using the phrase '*evidence-based practice*', and limited to '*nursing*', revealed 8740 relevant articles. From this alone it is safe to say there has been an explosion of interest in this area.

Implicit in such discussions is the message that healthcare, wherever it is delivered, must be based on good, sound evidence. In days gone by, when asked why something was done in a particular way, a nurse's mantra was 'Sister says so' or 'We've always done it this way'. It has been suggested that historically clinical issues have been based on a form of craft-based knowledge or 'habit, intuition and sometimes plain old guessing' (Gawande, 2003: 7). This is no longer sufficient and there is an expectation that strong evidence must underpin nurses' practice. Mantzoukas (2007) has identified that EBP is central to the notion of best practice, nurse accountability and the need to ensure that nursing activities are transparent and safe.

Whilst the importance of research in the delivery of nursing care has always been emphasised, the idea of evidence-based practice is seen as focusing the minds of those involved in care delivery on the use of appropriate evidence. There is also a perceived lack of enthusiasm in relation to the implementation of nursing research. Glasziou and Haynes (2005) proposed that some research, essential to the delivery of quality of care, will go unrecognised for years and suggested the major barriers to using evidence are time, effort and the skills involved in accessing information from the myriad of data available. EBP is seen as a way of addressing this.

Ingersoll (2000) has also argued that focusing EBP on care delivery reflects the differences between it and research. Research concentrates on knowledge discovery whereas in EBP the application of knowledge is central. In addition she has suggested that whilst this emphasis on EBP is a welcome initiative, the wholesale 'lifting' of approaches and methodologies from another discipline such as medicine is not. Nurses need to make sure that the evidence used is relevant to the practice of nursing. There is a range of such evidence that can inform practice – personal experience and reflection literature, research, policy, guidelines, clinical expertise and audit (Dale, 2005) – all of which have their place within EBP and will be explored further in the various chapters of this book.

So what is EBP?

At its simplest, EBP is about good practice and improving the quality of care, however achieving this is a complex undertaking. Various definitions are available (see Box 1.1). French (1999) suggested that the common threads of these definitions presented EBP as:

- based on problems identified from the practitioner's area of practice;
- a combining of best evidence and professional expertise and an integration of this into current practice;
- about ensuring patients receive quality care, being part of quality improvement processes;
- about collaboration and requiring a team approach.

Box 1.1   Definition of EBP

RCN (1996: 3): 'doing the right thing in the right way for the right patient at the right time'.

Pearson et al. (2007:14) 'the melding of individual clinical judgement and expertise with the best available external evidence to generate the kind of practice that is most likely to lead to a positive outcome for a client or patient.'

> Ingersoll (2000: 152): 'the conscientious, explicit and judicious use of theory-derived, research-based information in making decisions about care delivery to individuals or groups of patients and in consideration of individual needs and preferences'.
>
> Dale (2005: 49): EBP involves 'the nurse making conscious judgements about available evidence'.
>
> Cullum et al. (2008: 2): evidence-based nursing is 'the application of valid, relevant, research-based information in nurse decision making'.

Scott and McSherry (2008) support French's assertion, proposing the key elements of EBP are that it is a theory-driven process which involves the use, evaluation and application of research; identification of best evidence; evaluation of care; problem solving; decision making; clinical expertise; and requires patient involvement.

Considering Scott and McSherry (2008) and French (1999) identified key features it is fair to say that the critical elements of EBP can be represented as:

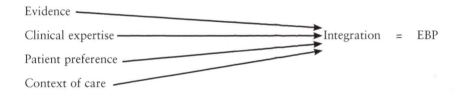

Where did the idea of EBP come from?

Professor Archie Cochrane, a British epidemiologist, is most frequently credited with starting the EBP movement. In his book *Effectiveness and Efficiency: Random Reflections on the Health Service* (Cochrane, 1972) he criticised the medical profession for not using appropriate evidence to guide and direct medical practice and challenged medicine to produce an evidence base. He argued there was a need to ensure treatment was delivered in the most effective manner and to ensure that available evidence was used in a consistent way.

When Cochrane talked of evidence, he meant randomised control trials (RCTs), which he viewed as providing the most reliable evidence on which to base medical care. RCTs are a form of research which uses experimental designs to identify the effectiveness of interventions. The use of systematic reviews, which summarise the findings of a number of RCTs looking at similar areas of interest, was suggested as the 'gold standard' of the scientific evidence on which to base medical interventions.

The medical profession responded to Cochrane's challenge by creating the Cochrane Centre for systematic reviews, which opened in 1992 in Oxford. The Cochrane Collaboration was founded in 1993, consisting of international review groups (currently encompassing more than 28,000 people in over 100 countries) covering a range of clinical areas and producing systematic reviews. These reviews are published electronically, updated regularly and there are now over 4600 of these available.

Activity

Visit the Cochrane Collaboration website (www.cochrane.org) and identify one systematic review abstract that would be of interest in relation to your current clinical environment.

Other collaborations have emerged since this time. For example, the Joanna Briggs Institute (JBI) – an international EBP collaboration made up of over 70 centres – was established in Australia in 1996. Its aim is to evaluate evidence from a wide range of sources, including all research methodologies, clinical experience and expertise. The JBI has identified three activities central to its role in relation to EBP:

- evidence synthesis – the bringing together of evidence in the form of systematic reviews;
- evidence transfer – targeting the evidence at clinical areas in forms that are easily accessible, such as 'best practice' information;
- evidence utilisation – providing tools that will enable evidence to be used and embedded in practice, such as audit tools.

Activity

Visit the JBI website (www.joannabriggs.edu.au) and find a best practice sheet relevant to your most recent practice experience. Read the sheet and consider what implications this might have for your own clinical practice.

The idea for **evidence-based medicine** (EBM) grew out of Cochrane's work. McMaster Medical School in Canada is credited with coining the term in 1980 to describe a particular learning approach used in the school. This approach had four steps – formulating a question related to a clinical problem; searching the literature for relevant information; critically appraising the literature; and using the findings to direct clinical practice (Peile, 2004).

Sackett et al. (1996: 71) defined evidence-based medicine as 'the conscientious, explicit and judicious use of current best evidence in making decisions about the care of individual patients'. Whilst the underpinning principles of EBM were hotly debated, the medical profession in general began to accept the idea, and 1995 saw the first issue of the journal *Evidence-Based Medicine for Primary Care and Internal Medicine*, published by the British Medical Journal Group. In 2007 EBM was identified as one of 15 major milestones in the development of medical practice since 1840 (BMJ, 2007). Nursing, emulating its medical colleagues, began to explore the notion of basing its practice on reliable sources of evidence, which resulted in the journal *Evidence-Based Nursing* appearing in 1998.

Social and political drivers of EBP

Scott and McSherry (2008) suggested a number of social and political factors facilitated the emergence of the emphasis on evidence at this time. The availability of 'knowledge' via the internet and other sources brought into being 'expert patients' – well-educated and informed individuals who accessed information relating to health and illness. Expectations of these expert patients were that healthcare professions would be aware of and use up-to-date information/research in their delivery of care and treatment. There was no longer a willingness simply to accept treatment or care purely on the advice of a doctor or nurse.

The concept of EBP was also seen as attractive by governments and health service administrators because of its potential to provide cost-effective care that was also seen as clinically effective (McSherry et al., 2006). In the mid-1990s the UK government of the day identified that quality assurance was to be placed at the forefront of the NHS modernisation agenda. Two White Papers – *The New NHS: Modern and Dependable* (Department of Health [DH], 1997) and *A First Class Service: Quality in the New NHS* (DH, 1998) – outlined the plans for promoting **clinical effectiveness** and introducing **clinical governance**: these gave systems to ensure quality improvement mechanisms were adopted at all levels of healthcare provision. Central to clinical governance were concepts of risk management and promoting clinical excellence. (See Figure 1.1 for an outline of the clinical governance framework.)

Clinical effectiveness was defined by the NHS Executive (1996) as 'the extent to which specific clinical interventions when deployed in the field for a particular patient or population, do what they are intended to do, that is maintain and improve health and secure the greatest possible health gain'. This definition continues to underpin the current DH approach to clinical effectiveness (DH, 2007a), with the various stages of the process being identified as:

- the development of best practice guidelines;
- the transfer of knowledge into practice through education, audit and practice development;
- the evaluation of the impact of guidelines through audit and patient feedback.

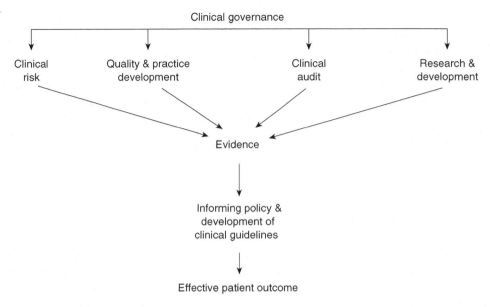

Figure 1.1   Representation of the elements of clinical governance

Put simply, clinical effectiveness can be seen as identifying appropriate evidence in the form of research, clinical guidelines, systematic reviews and national standards; changing practice to include this evidence; evaluating the impact of any change and making the necessary adjustments through the use of clinical audit and patient feedback/service evaluation. Table 1.1 provides an overview of the key aspects of research, **clinical audit** and **service evaluation**.

Two organisations were created aimed at promoting an evidence-based approach to health care, which are known today as the National Institute for Health and Clinical Excellence (NICE) and the Care Quality Commission (CQC). These bodies provided guidance for healthcare managers and practitioners and were charged with ensuring this guidance is followed in England and Wales. In Scotland the Health Technology Board fulfils a similar purpose. Clinical governance was introduced to ensure healthcare was both efficient and effective; healthcare professionals were expected to show EBP supported all aspects of care delivery and service developments. It was hoped that the introduction of these measures would result in a shift in organisational culture from one that was reactive, responding as issues arise, to one with a proactive ethos, where the healthcare offered is known to be effective and therefore avoids unforeseen outcomes.

NICE and the now CQC have continued to develop strategies to promote clinical effectiveness. The former through initiatives such as 'How to ...' guides, quality standards and supporting a resource known as 'NHS Evidence'. The NHS Evidence site provides access to various forms of evidence which may be of use in clinical practice and provides examples of best practice. The CQC was charged with ensuring the safety and quality of care through inspection and assessment of all healthcare provision. The NHS Institute for Innovation and Improvement was set up in 2006 with a remit to support the implementation of service improvement initiatives within the NHS.

Table 1.1 Research, audit and service evaluation

Research	Service evaluations*	Clinical audit
The attempt to derive generalisable new knowledge including studies that aim to generate hypotheses as well as studies that aim to test them	Designed and conducted solely to define or judge current care	Designed and conducted to produce information to inform delivery of best care
Quantitative research – designed to test a hypothesis. Qualitative research – identifies/explores themes following established methodologies	Designed to answer: 'What standard does this service achieve?'	Designed to answer: 'Does this service reach a predetermined standard?'
Addresses clearly defined questions, aims and objectives	Measures a current service without reference to a standard	Measures against a standard
Quantitative research – may involve evaluating or comparing interventions, particularly new ones Qualitative research – usually involves studying how intervention and relationships are experienced	Involves an intervention in use only. The choice of treatment is that of the clinician and patient according to guidance, professional standards and/ or patient preferences	Involves an intervention in use only. The choice of treatment is that of the clinician and patient according to guidance, professional standards and/ or patient preferences
Usually involves collecting data that are additional to those for routine care but may include data collected routinely. May involve treatments, samples or investigations additional to routine care	Usually involves analysis of existing data but may include administration of interview or questionnaire	Usually involves analysis of existing data but may include administration of interview or questionnaire
Quantitative research – study design may involve allocating patients to intervention groups Qualitative research – uses a clearly defined sampling framework underpinned by conceptual or theoretical justifications	No allocation to intervention: the health professional and patient have chosen intervention before service evaluation	No allocation to intervention: the health professional and patient have chosen intervention before audit
May involve randomisation	No randomisation	No randomisation
Normally requires Research Ethics Committees review	Does not require REC review	Does not require REC review

*Service development and quality improvement may fall into this category

Source: Defining Research (Health Research Authority, 2009).

Activity

Identify one condition/disease you have come across recently in clinical practice (e.g. dementia). Visit the NICE website (www.nice.org.uk) and locate the NICE guidance and NHS evidence available in relation to your chosen condition/disease.

Concerns about EBP

Evidence-based approaches are not without their problems; as Davies et al. (2007: 26) identified it has both 'enthusiastic supporters and vociferous detractors'. Melnyk and Fineout-Overholt (2005) suggested that EBP is viewed by many as simply another term for research utilisation. It has also been argued elsewhere that the value of research has been over-emphasised to the detriment of clinical judgement and person-centred approaches, while others point to a lack of evidence to support the notion that EBP improves health outcomes.

Kitson (2002) has pointed to an inherent tension between EBP and person-centred approaches. She has argued that clinical expertise is vital in ensuring that patients' experiences and needs are not sidelined in the pursuit of 'best evidence' in the form of research findings and the development of generalised clinical guidelines. Some individuals have suggested that such broad general principles are not applicable to certain aspects of care. Davies et al. (2007) suggested that practitioners often feel that an over-emphasis on EBP inhibits their ability to provide individualised care. Melnyk and Fineout-Overholt (2005) have identified this as a 'cookbook' approach, where a general recipe is followed with no consideration for the specific needs or preferences of individuals. There are concerns also around the ability to have a consensus in relation to the various interpretations available when translating evidence into guidelines and the relevance of these for individual areas of practice. There are also issues related to the updating of evidence and the ability to ensure that the information gathered is current. However, DiCenso et al. (2008) argue that as clinical expertise and decision-making processes are central to EBP, in considering the use of general guidelines both of these processes must be used in the same way with any form of evidence including guidance.

However, Brady and Lewin (2007) identify that whilst the idea of clinical expertise is readily accepted by most experienced nurses, the majority of those same nurses are often unaware of the latest research in their area of practice. Nurses are generally presented as relying on intuition, tradition and local policies/procedures to guide their practice. Stevens (2004) proposed that healthcare providers frequently do not use current knowledge for a number of reasons, not least of these being the rapidly growing and changing body of research, some of which is difficult to apply to practice directly. As the aim of EBP is to deliver high quality care, nurses need to have an understanding of what the exact elements of EBP are and to then develop the necessary skills and knowledge to enable them to carry this out.

French (1999) suggested that as EBP is so closely linked with EBM and its preference for certain types of evidence, there is a danger that this promotes the use of medical knowledge over other forms and therefore leads to a medicalisation of healthcare environments to the detriment of other disciplines. Best evidence in the medical context is often taken to mean quantitative research findings – as identified above in the form of RCTs. Some have questioned its compatibility with nursing and the other health professions, suggesting instead the use of a more open approach. Dale (2005) proposed that this issue has the potential to create interprofessional conflict, as that which nursing may count as appropriate evidence on which to base practice may be somewhat different from that of the medical profession.

What skills are needed?

EBP is often represented as a process that has a number of steps within it. Sackett et al. (2000) have suggested a four-step model:

1   Ask an answerable question.
2   Find the appropriate evidence.
3   Critically appraise that evidence.
4   Apply the evidence to the patient, giving consideration to the individual needs, presentation and context.

JBI has a similar model with six steps – see Box 1.2.

Box 1.2   JBI model of EBP

- Search for evidence.
- Appraise evidence.
- Summarise evidence.
- Utilise.
- Embed.
- Evaluate impact.

Aas and Alexanderson (2011) suggested that the various models have common aspects and from these have identified a 'Five A' step process (see Table 1.2).

Table 1.2   'Five A' steps to EBP

- Assess – identify a problem and the need for further information
- Ask – generate the question to be answered
- Acquire – find the relevant evidence
- Appraise – critically appraise the evidence and its relevance to practice context
- Apply – identify how best to apply the evidence to the practice setting

There are common themes that run through all these models which would suggest there is a need to develop particular skills and knowledge related to:

- the ability to identify what counts as appropriate evidence;
- forming a question to enable you to find evidence for consideration;
- developing a search strategy;

- finding the evidence;
- critically appraising the evidence;
- drawing on clinical expertise;
- issues concerned with patient preference;
- application to the context of care delivery;
- putting the evidence into practice.

Why does your practice need to be evidence-based

As Craig and Pearson (2007) have already identified, few in the healthcare professions would disagree with the ideas underpinning EBP – namely, that care should be of the highest standard and delivered in the most effective way. Indeed practising without any 'evidence' to guide our actions amounts to little more than providing care that is based on trial and error, which none of us would advocate. However, as identified above, care is not always based on the best evidence, with Greenhalgh (2006) suggesting that many of the decisions made in healthcare are based on four main sources of information:

1 *Anecdotal information.* Here it is considered that 'it worked in situation X so it must be appropriate to (the similar) situation Y'. However, as Greenhalgh points out, while situations may seem very similar, patient responses are often very different.
2 *Press cuttings information.* Here changes are made to practice in response to reading one article or editorial, without critically appraising and considering the applicability of those results to the specific setting.
3 *Consensus statements.* Here a group of 'experts' will identify the best approaches based on their experiences/beliefs. Whilst clinical expertise does have a place in EBP, it does not operate without some problems. For example, clinical wisdom once held (and to a certain extent still does hold) that bed rest was the most appropriate form of treatment for acute lower back pain. However, research in 1986 demonstrated that this is potentially harmful.
4 *Cost minimisation.* Here the limited resources available within a healthcare setting will often result in choosing the cheapest option in an effort to spread resources as widely as possible. However, EBP can ensure the most effective use of limited and pressurised resources. Whilst certain types of care may appear more expensive on the surface, if these prove more effective, they may turn out to be cheaper in the long run.

Perhaps part of the problem related to nursing developing an EBP ethos is that nursing is often considered as more of an art than a science and as such certain types of evidence are valued above others, such as expert opinion and practice experience. However, Polit and Beck (2008: 4) identified that any nursing action must be 'clinically appropriate, cost effective and result in a positive outcome for clients'. The complexity of healthcare, and the uncertainty of people's responses to and experiences of different types of interventions, require that a full consideration is given to all the available evidence.

Patients are likely to know a great deal about their own health needs and to expect health professionals to base care decisions on the most up-to-date and clinically relevant information. There is also an expectation that professionals will be able to comment in an informed way on any research reported in the media and identify its relevance to and appropriateness for an individual's health needs. Miller and Forrest (2001) proposed that the ability to ensure that a professional's knowledge and skills remain current increases their professional credibility; allows them to be an important source of information to those in their care as well as colleagues; and enables all professionals involved in care delivery to make well-informed decisions. It has also been suggested that EBP provides the framework by which such demands may be met and can foster a lifelong learning approach – an essential requirement in the health professions if staff are to remain effective in rapidly changing healthcare environments.

EBP Activity

Consider the list of skills identified above as associated with EBP (listed on p. 11). Choose three areas which you feel you have most difficulty with and undertake a SWOT analysis in relation to each one using the grid in Appendix 1.

Summary

- EBP is a global phenomenon which promotes the idea of best practice, clinical effectiveness and quality care and involves an integration of evidence, clinical expertise, patient preferences and the clinical context of care delivery to inform clinical decision making.
- EBP focuses on critically appraising evidence to support care delivery rather than on research to discover new knowledge.
- The emergence of the expert patient has given rise to the need for health professionals to ensure they are up-to-date and their care based on best evidence available.
- Government initiatives have promoted EBP as a way of providing both clinically effective and cost-effective healthcare.
- Various steps are associated with the EBP process – forming a question; finding evidence; critically appraising the evidence; integration of evidence into practice.
- The knowledge and skills associated with EBP are an essential component of nursing practice.

Further reading

Cranston, M. (2002) 'Clinical effectiveness and evidence-based practice', *Nursing Standard*, 16(24): 39–43. Provides a concise account of the meaning of clinical governance, the place of clinical effectiveness within this concept and the drive towards EBP.

Rycroft-Malone, J., Seers, K., Titchen, A., Harvey, G., Kitson, A. and McCormack, B. (2004) 'What counts as evidence in evidence-based practice?', *Journal of Advanced Nursing*, 47(1): 81–90. This article gives a clear overview of the evidence-based movement and issues related to the nature of evidence.

E-resources

Cochrane Collaboration: promotes, supports and prepares systematic reviews, mainly in relation to effectiveness. www.cochrane.org/

Joanna Briggs Institute: promotes evidence-based healthcare through systematic reviews and a range of resources aimed at promoting evidence synthesis, transfer and utilisation. www.joannabriggs.edu.au

National Institute for Health and Clinical Excellence: provides guidance and other products to enable and support health professionals deliver evidence-based care. www.nice.org.uk

2

The Nature of Knowledge, Evidence and How to Ask the Right Questions

Learning Outcomes

By the end of the chapter you will be able to:

- discuss the nature of knowledge;
- identify what is meant by 'evidence';
- form a question to allow identification and selection of best evidence;
- understand the use of the PICO framework in forming research questions.

Introduction

It is suggested that humans have a basic need for knowledge and a thirst to know how things work and why things happen. Parahoo (1997) proposed that knowledge is essential for human survival, and central to decision making about daily life and achieving change in both people and the environment in which they live. Prior to the 18th century much of people's understanding of the world and how it worked was based on beliefs related to superstitions and organised religions. However, the 18th century ushered in what we know as the era of 'Enlightenment' and the 'Age of Reason' which promoted different ways of thinking and knowing the world. The work of individuals known as 'encyclopaedists' (generally the leading philosophers of the day) and the publication of the *Encyclopedie* in the period from 1751 to 1772 together advocated scientific knowledge. This type of knowledge influenced thinking about the nature of humans and their ways of understanding the world and from this came an opening of the debate about what is knowledge and how humans can 'know' things.

Knowledge and evidence are inextricably linked – evidence provides support to the usefulness of certain types of knowledge and knowledge gives reason and value to different forms of evidence. Therefore as with knowledge there are many different forms of evidence, each of which will be valued in different ways in different contexts. This chapter will consider the issues surrounding the nature of knowledge, the different forms of evidence and how it is possible to identify what it is that you need to know in order to ensure your practice is evidence-based.

Nature of knowledge

Knowledge can be defined as 'the facts or experiences known by a person or group of people; specific information about a subject' (Collins Dictionary, 1998). Knowledge is broadly categorised into two types – **propositional** and **non-propositional**. Propositional or codified knowledge is said to be public knowledge and is often given a formal status by its inclusion in educational programmes. Non-propositional knowledge is personal knowledge linked to experience, and is described by Eraut (2000) as a 'cognitive resource' – a way of making sense of things – that someone brings to any given situation to help them think and act. It is often linked to '**tacit**' knowledge. This is knowledge which is often difficult to put into words. For instance, you may know how to ride a bike and know how you learnt to do it, but may not be able to describe critical aspects, such as how you keep your balance.

In considering where knowledge comes from Kerlinger (1973) identifies three sources – **tenacity, authority** and **a priori**. Tenacity relates to knowledge that is believed simply because it has always been held as the truth. Authority relates to knowledge which comes from a source or person viewed as being authoritative and therefore must be true. A priori knowing relates to reasoning processes, where it is reasonable to consider something to be true. It is suggested that all three sources of knowledge are viewed as being objective in nature and not based on a person's subjective view of the world (see Box 2.1 for examples of these types of knowledge).

Box 2.1   Example of three sources of knowledge

An individual with a cold knows that taking cough mixture will soothe their cough. If asked how they know this they might answer:

- 'because I know it does' – tenacity;
- 'because my mother told me it does' – authority;
- 'because it stands to reason that cough medicine will soothe a cough' – a priori.

It has been suggested that in relation to clinical decision making there are four forms of knowledge available to practitioners – superstition, folk lore, craft and science (Justice, 2010). Superstition is similar to tenacity in that it is a belief which has no rational basis, such as the belief that bad things always happen in threes. Folk lore relates more to a pattern of beliefs put forward at an earlier time which are slow to be replaced by other, more feasible explanations for behaviours, such as the belief that the cycles of the moon affect the behaviour of people with mental health problems. Craft-based knowledge is seen most commonly as being practice-based knowledge – gained through clinical experience and drawing on personal judgement and intuition. However there may well be a theoretical aspect, often gained during initial professional education. Science is a broad term relating to the ways of understanding the world. It is frequently thought to have a uniform definition; however, as will be discussed below, there are different views as to what can be deemed 'scientific knowledge'.

Activity

Think about recent experiences in practice. Can you identify examples of knowledge which are based on tenacity, authority and a priori sources and also those that appear to have their basis in superstition, folk lore and craft knowledge?

Scientific knowledge

The term **science** comes from the Latin word *scietia*, meaning knowledge. Such knowledge has traditionally been seen as being based on observation, experiment and measurement (Mason and Whitehead, 2003). Scientific knowledge is usually generated either through **deductive** or **inductive** reasoning (Speziale and Carpenter, 2007). Deductive reasoning is said to move from the general to the particular, while inductive goes from the particular to the general. With deductive reasoning the nurse would start with a **hypothesis** which she or he would then seek to prove. A hypothesis is a simple statement that identifies a cause and effect relationship between two things – if I do X then Y is likely to happen. For example, in relation to considering the use of wound dressings (the general issue) the nurse might consider that one form of dressing (the particular) is more effective than another. The hypothesis might be that *wound dressing A will promote more rapid wound healing than dressing B*. In inductive reasoning, a nurse might start by considering somebody's experience of leg ulcers (a specific issue); she or he could then interview various people who have the condition, asking them about their experiences. Once a number of views have been collected it is possible to draw conclusions and a general theory of the experience could then be developed.

Deductive reasoning is often associated with **positivism**, the idea that reality is ordered, regular, can be studied objectively and quantified. A basic component of positivism is **empiricism**, where it is proposed that only that which can be observed can be called fact or truth. Originally such observation was intended to mean observation by human senses – sight, touch and so on. However, over time this has been expanded to include indirect observation through the use of specific tools designed to help a scientist observe and record phenomena. So whereas the study of personality could be viewed as impossible because you can't see it, the development of a personality inventory provides a tool that the scientist can use to study it empirically. The idea of 'cause and effect' is also important in empiricism – if I do this (cause) then this (effect) will happen – so for example if dressing X is used (cause) the wound will heal more quickly (effect). Empiricism is often described as reductionist, which relates to the breaking down of areas of interest into small parts rather than considering the whole.

Inductive reasoning is linked with **interpretivism,** an alternative to positivism based on the belief that humans are actively involved in constructing their understanding of the world. It is proposed that individuals constantly strive to understand what is happening in their environment and interpret action and interaction in an effort to make sense of their experiences. From this perspective, it is proposed that there are a range of views of the world and ways of understanding, depending on the interpretation people give to their experiences. Rather than adopting reductionist approaches and identifying cause and effect, interpretivism is seen as considering the whole, exploring all the meanings and seeking a full as possible understanding of phenomena.

As can be seen from above, philosophical positions are adopted about the nature of the world, what can be known and how to gather this knowledge. These philosophical positions are known as **paradigms,** a term created by Kuhn (1970). A paradigm is a set of logically connected ideas which guide the way in which research can be conducted – the methods used, the form of data collected and how that data are analysed. Two paradigms are generally accepted as being present in research – qualitative and quantitative – based on two different and sometimes competing ways of discovering the world. Qualitative research is concerned with exploring the meanings people attach to experiences and generating theories, whereas quantitative is focused on generating data to prove or disprove theories. The paradigms are reflected in the way data are collected – qualitative data tend to be in the form of words, what people say about their experiences; quantitative data are presented in the form of numbers providing a basis for statistical analysis. Examples of how research into the same general area might look are given in Table 2.1.

Table 2.1   Examples of research questions

An investigation of anxiety in patients	
What is the nature of anxiety in patients? What sorts of things provoke anxiety and what is the relationship between them?	Are patients who are supplied with information less anxious than those who are not?
This is a qualitative approach ... the question is a 'what IS this?' type. Suggests an inductive approach, moving from the specific to the general.	This requires a quantitative approach. Suggests a cause and effect relationship and then tests it.

Table 2.2 Differences between quantitative and qualitative research

Quantitative	Qualitative
Scientific principles	Understanding/meaning of events
Moves from theory to data	Moves from data to theory
Identification of causal relationships between data	A close understanding of the research context
Collection of adequate amount of data	Collection of 'rich/deep' data
Application of controls to ensure validity	Seeks to address all aspects of the issues
Highly structured	Flexible structure allowing for changes in emphasis
Objectivity	Researcher as part of the process
Acceptance/rejection of hypothesis/laws	Generation of theory

Quantitative methods include randomised control trials (RCTs), experimental designs and involve statistical analysis of data. Qualitative enquiry includes phenomenology, ethnography, action research and grounded theory and generally involves interviews and observation, although some forms may incorporate aspects of statistical analysis. Table 2.2 provides a brief summary of the difference between qualitative and quantitative approaches. Issues related to the research approaches are discussed in further detail in Chapters 7 and 8.

Nursing knowledge

There is much debate as to what constitutes nursing knowledge. Knowledge plays a complex role in professions, often being seen as a defining trait. Schon (1987) suggested there is a hierarchy of knowledge in professions:

- basic science;
- applied science;
- technical skills of everyday practice.

He also suggested that professions' status is dependent on this hierarchy, that the closer a professional knowledge base is to basic science the higher the status. Nursing has tried for many years to establish a defined scientific knowledge base. Huntington and Gilmour (2001) stated that nursing has traditionally focused on empirical approaches to knowledge generation and has used these to explain the nature of nursing practice. The development of this knowledge has been influenced by other disciplines such as medicine, psychology and sociology. Although for a number of years scientific knowledge has been accepted as superior to other forms, more recently this has been challenged and there is a growing belief that other forms of knowledge are essential in the practice of nursing.

Carper (1978) was one of the first people to provide a framework through which the patterns of knowing in nursing could be considered. She identified four types of nursing knowledge – *empirical, personal, aesthetic* and *ethical* – and suggested that no one form of knowledge is superior to the other, instead each was essential to the practice of nursing. Empirical knowledge is seen as the theoretical and research-based knowledge which is generated through systematic investigation and observation. This may also be knowledge generated by other disciplines which can be seen as either a theory underpinning practice (such as anatomy and physiology) or a theory translated for use in nursing in a unique way (as with applied sciences such as psychology). Chinn and Kramer (2004) added the development of nursing theory to the concept of empirical knowledge, particularly in relation to interpretive research approaches such as phenomenology.

Personal knowledge relates to the individual nurse's experience of the world generally and nursing specifically. It encompasses that person's beliefs, values, perception and level of self-awareness. In many ways it resembles reflective practice, as implicit within this is the ability to know yourself and how this influences your practice. The emotional aspects of nursing require nurses to consider how and why they respond to certain situations in certain ways to ensure the care they deliver is appropriate and compassionate. This type of knowledge is something that is seen as changing over time and having direct implications on the type and form of interactions that occur between nurses and patients.

Aesthetic knowledge is described as that knowledge which underpins the 'art' of nursing. It can be seen as a bringing together of the manual, technical and intellectual skills aspects of nursing, particularly in nurse and patient interactions. This type of knowledge is often linked to expert practice and the ability to assist individuals in coping with health issues in a positive way.

Finally ethical knowledge is seen as focusing on what is right, appropriate and moral: it relates to the judgements to be made in relation to nursing actions. It is also related to codes of conduct, procedural guidelines and the philosophical principles that underpin nursing.

Activity

Reflect on a recent clinical placement. Can you identify specific incidents where you used Carper's four types of knowledge?

Table 2.3 gives examples of activities associated with the different types of knowledge identified by Carper.

Intuition is an area that has been the subject of much debate, with what is termed **intuitive knowledge** being seen by many as an important aspect of nursing practice. Intuition can be defined as the 'instant understanding of knowledge without evidence of sensible thought' (Billay et al., 2007: 147) and is often considered to

Table 2.3 Examples of activities associated with different types of knowledge

Knowledge	Example
Empirical	Biological sciences knowledge to understand blood pressure readings
	Psychology theory in relation to phobias to understand a patient's fear of injections/needles
Personal	'Therapeutic use of self' in understanding a person's response when given 'bad news'
	Interpersonal relationships, therapeutic relationships
Ethical	Code of conduct
	Confidentiality
Aesthetic	Communicating with a patient in a caring and appropriate way before giving an injection
	Recognising the individual needs of a person when helping them with personal hygiene

be a form of tacit knowledge. It is the moment when you 'know' that something is going to happen, or reach a conclusion, without being aware of thinking in a rational and logical way to arrive at that point. In considering the nature of intuition in professional practice, Benner (1984) suggested that a form of practice knowledge or 'expertise' exists which is part of expert practice. Here a nurse draws on all their empirical and personal knowledge to reach a conclusion, without being aware of processing the information. See Box 2.2 for an example. Benner differentiates between practical and theoretical knowledge suggesting that the former relates to 'knowing how' and related to skills and the latter to 'knowing that', which is concerned with the generation of theory and scientific knowledge. However, she also suggested that in nursing, as expertise develops, a form of practice knowledge is apparent that 'side steps' the logical reasoning processes associated with science. Extending the knowing how of practice through practice experience can lead to knowledge that appears to be available to the person without the aid of analytical process, but which nevertheless is valid.

Box 2.2 Example of expert knowledge (Benner, 1984: 32)

An extract from an interview with a nurse who worked in the psychiatric setting for 15 years:

> When I say to a doctor 'this patient is psychotic', I don't always know how to legitimize that statement. But I am never wrong. Because I know psychosis from inside out. And I feel that, and I know it, and I trust it. I don't care if nothing else is happening, I still really know that. It's like the feeling another nurse described in the small group interview today, when she said about the patient 'she just isn't right.'

Other forms of knowing have been added to Carper's original work. For example Mullhall (1993) put forward the idea of 'unknowing', proposing that nurses needed to make deliberate attempts to be open to new ideas and ways of thinking; seeing this as a step in building knowledge and a deeper understanding of individual practice experiences. Sociopolitical knowledge was included by White (1995). Here political awareness, cultural diversity and public health agendas are seen as essential aspects of knowing, enabling nursing to see their practice in a broader arena. Chinn and Kramer (2008) proposed 'emancipatory knowledge': an awareness of social inequalities and their implication for health, including a political awareness, the need for social change and methods to bring this about.

What constitutes evidence?

The dictionary definition of evidence is 'grounds for belief or disbelief; data on which to base proof or establish truth or falsehood' (Collins Dictionary, 1998). Pearson (2005) proposed in healthcare that it is 'data or information used to decide whether or not a claim or view should be trusted'. What exactly constitutes evidence in EBP is still hotly debated. Thomas (2004) suggested that evidence is information that is seen as relevant to how to provide care and beliefs about health and illness. Various hierarchies of evidence have been generated which clearly place quantitative findings from systematic reviews of RCTs at the top of the hierarchy, often qualitative research findings are not included within these hierarchies at all (see Box 2.3 for an example of a hierarchy). This preference for one form of evidence over another perhaps comes from the Cochrane Collaboration, which focused on the effectiveness of interventions for which RCTs are ideally suited and also on the dominance of the positivist paradigm in terms of research approaches.

Box 2.3   An example of a hierarchy of evidence

1 Systematic reviews of RCTs.

2 Well-designed RCTs.

3 Other types of experimental studies – pre-post test, cohort, time series.

4 Non-experimental studies.

5 Descriptive studies, expert committee reports.

However there is a growing body of literature that hotly contests the placing of RCT methods at the top of the hierarchy. Scott and McSherry (2008) suggested that RCTs are not always the most pertinent approach to certain aspects of nursing care.

Porter and O'Halloran (2012) support this assertion and identified that RCTs do not provide the best evidence for the complex systems in which healthcare is delivered. Different types of research questions require different forms of study. Therefore the most appropriate form of evidence is that which relates to the question being asked – 'horse for courses' as Petticrew and Roberts (2003) put it.

Nursing has long recognised that its practice is based on multiple ways of knowing and much of nursing's activities do not fit easily with an RCT approach. The advocating of one type of evidence as superior to another is not helpful in providing evidence on which to base practice in a profession as multifaceted and complex as nursing. It is suggested that perhaps it is more appropriate to acknowledge the possibility of multiple hierarchies, depending on the object or issue under consideration. Nairn (2012: 14) proposed 'there is one world, but multiple ways of examining that world'.

The Joanna Briggs Institute (JBI) supports the idea of there being a range of issues that need to be considered in healthcare, and that different forms of evidence are needed. They suggest that evidence generally falls into four areas:

1   Evidence of feasibility – whether something is practical/practicable physically, culturally or financially. In this situation one type of treatment might be the most effective, but financially unaffordable. For example the cost of certain drugs means they are not used in certain healthcare systems. Types of evidence to support this would probably be economic and policy research.
2   Evidence of appropriateness – whether a particular intervention fits with the context in which it is to be given. For example blood transfusion within certain religious groups might not be an appropriate form of treatment. Research considering ethical and philosophical issues would be of use here.
3   Evidence of meaningfulness – how interventions/activities are experienced by individuals. For example, the patients' experiences of or beliefs about fertility treatment might influence how services are organised. Interpretive research in the form of phenomenology, ethnology or grounded theory would be of interest in this area.
4   Evidence of effectiveness – whether one treatment is better than another or the usual intervention. RCTs and cohort studies would be of use here.

Rycroft-Malone et al. (2004a) suggested there are four types of evidence on which nurses can base their practice:

1   Research.
2   Clinical experience.
3   Service user/carer perspectives.
4   Local context.

They went on to identify that the challenge is in knowing how to integrate these four types of evidence in a robust and patient-centred way.

Ensuring the robustness of evidence related to clinical experience requires the gathering and documenting of this experience in a systematic manner, allowing for individual and group reflection and cross-checking. Portfolios and clinical supervision are methods which can enhance the validity of this type of evidence and these are explored further in Chapter 11.

Incorporating sources of evidence from service users and carers into the delivery of care has a long tradition within nursing and underpins the ethos of holistic care. This aspect is explored further in Chapter 3, however it has to be said that this source of evidence has its own inherent complexities and can be challenging. When research findings promoting the view that a specific form of intervention is most appropriate (for example the use of a particular medication in managing mental health problems) are at odds with the service user's experience (the medication has specific side effects that make the person unwilling to take it), the clinical expertise of the nurse is essential in identifying the most appropriate course of action.

Institutional cultures, social and professional networks, evaluations such as 360 degree feedback and local/national policies are some of the forms of evidence found in the local setting (Rycroft-Malone et al., 2004a). Other relevant local evidence includes audits and individual patient preferences and service evaluations.

There are also some 'ready made' forms of evidence available, where best evidence has been collected and summarised for use by healthcare professionals. Clinical Knowledge Summaries is an example of this type of resource. This is an online collection of concise summaries of available evidence, providing recommendations on how to manage commonly encountered clinical situations in primary care settings (www.cks.library.nhs.uk).

A relatively new initiative in EBP is that of **care bundles**. Here elements of best practice evidence (usually between three and five) are grouped together in relation to a particular condition, treatment and/or procedure. These elements are ones that are generally used in practice but not necessarily applied in the same way or combination to all appropriate patients. Care bundles 'tie' together these elements into a unit that is delivered to every patient in the same way. Dawson and Endacott (2011) identified that combining elements in this way has a more positive impact on treatment outcomes than any single one element. They suggested that care bundles appear to be more effective than clinical guidelines in improving possible outcomes, as the former are seen as mandatory whilst the latter are often viewed as purely advisory.

Care bundles were originally developed in 2002 at the Johns Hopkins University in the US in relation to critical care environments. It was found that using four interventions with patients on ventilators significantly reduced length of stay and number of ventilator days. Care bundles have been developed in a number of areas, such as infection control, and are advocated by the Department of Health as a tool for high impact change. However the Institute for Healthcare Improvement (2012) warns against an ad hoc approach to bringing elements of care together, stressing that the strength of the bundles lies in the underpinning science, the way it is delivered and a consistency in its application.

Questions

Having identified what counts as good evidence, the next task is to find the evidence. This requires the formulating of a relevant question, often considered the backbone of EBP. Ideas in relation to questions about practice can come from a range of situations, reflection on practice issues, audit outcomes and discussions between nurse, patients and/or other health professionals. Often such questions are broad and unfocused, but if appropriate answers are to be found then there is a need to be specific as what it is you want to know.

Activity

You are currently working in long-term care setting environment. Mary a 66-year-old patient in your care has fallen and fractured her femur. In discussion with the rest of the care staff it is identified that there have been a number of falls over the year that have resulted in fractured femurs. Someone remembers reading about 'hip protectors' as a method of reducing injuries. You have been asked to look for some evidence to help make decisions as to how to address the issues. Where would you start?

You might start by going online and 'Googling' the words 'fractured femur', but you are likely to quickly discover that this either produces thousands of hits or nothing at all. There is a need to focus your search to ensure that you get the relevant information whilst at the same time not missing vital pieces of information.

Stillwell et al. (2010a) identified there are two forms of questions that practitioners might ask – **background** and **foreground**. Background questions are generally broad and have two parts:

1 The question's stem – who, what, where, when, how, why?
2 The area of clinical interest.

A background question might look something like *What is the best way of treating depression?* There is a need to ask background questions, particularly for students and those new to an area of practice, in order to gain the knowledge and expertise needed in relation to a specific area. The problem with background questions is their broadness, which makes it difficult to find specific information, and searching for information is often done in a haphazard way – indeed you can easily end up looking in the wrong place.

Foreground questions ask about specific issues and are looking for particular knowledge. A foreground question might be something like *Which is more effect in treating depression – cognitive behavioural therapy or medication?*

It is essential that you formulate a foreground question containing all the key elements for consideration, before searching the literature in relation to a particular issue. The question will be central to ensuring that the search is not too broad, which in turn may result in retrieving an overwhelming amount of literature, or too narrow, resulting in key items being missed. There are a number of formats that can be used to help to create a search question; the most commonly used is **PICO** (see Table 2.4)

Table 2.4 Outline of PICO

Population	Intervention	Comparison	Outcome
Include 1 Disease/condition e.g. cancer, schizophrenia, Downs 2 Population (e.g. age) and setting (e.g. community)	Type of activity/ procedure/treatment or action, e.g. • Use of a specific assessment tool • Particular type of wound dressing • Using a particular approach such as cognitive behavioural therapy	Alternative activities or actions against which you compare your intervention. Sometimes this might be usual treatment	Results of a specified action. All possible outcomes are explored

As you can see from Table 2.4,

P = population and could be something like *adult males with depression.*
I = intervention and could be something like *cognitive behavioural therapy (CBT).*
C = comparison and could be something like *antidepressant medication.*
O = outcome and could be something like *raised mood.*

The PICO question would then be:

> In adult male service users diagnosed with depression is CBT more effective than antidepressants in raising mood?

In some instances the use of an extra letter such as T is added, which relates to the time frame over which the intervention would be observed, making PICOT. In the above question, for example, you could add '*over a period of 18 months*'. In other instances the letter S is added, giving the acronym PICOS, with the S = Study type providing the opportunity to limit the type of study you would want to include in your search of literature. In this case you might only want to consider RCTs.

Activity

Consider the above scenario about Mary, and apply the PICO principles. What question do you think would enable you to search for appropriate evidence?

It might look something like this:

> *In female adults over the age of 65 years, is the use of hip protection more effective than normal precautions in reducing the incidence of fractured femurs following a fall?*

The PICO framework tends to be most useful when asking 'effectiveness' questions and reflects the quantitative approach to research. However, it is less helpful for considering qualitative aspects of care such as patient experiences. The JBI offers an alternative formation – PICo:

Participants

phenomena of Interest

Context

If in relation to the above scenario you were actually interested in patients' experience of wearing hip protectors, the question in this instance might be:

> *In female adults over the age of 65 years (P), what is their experience of wearing hip protectors (I) in a hospital setting (Co)?*

Formulating questions in this way will enable you to focus on what is the real question that needs to be addressed and help you move on to the next stage of the process, searching for the evidence. The question will provide you with the key terms to be used in the search.

EBP Activity

Think about a recent clinical experience and identify a patient whose care you were closely involved with. Focusing on one clinical intervention you undertook in relation to this person (giving an injection, attending to hygiene needs, involvement of patients in recreational/ therapeutic activities), write a reflective account identifying:

(Continued)

(Continued)

1   What knowledge you were using during the intervention/activity, considering what areas of knowledge you felt most comfortable with and those that you need to develop further.
2   What evidence you used to direct how you organised your intervention/activity.
3   The questions you would ask if you wanted to find further evidence to support your practice in this area.

Summary

- Knowledge is broadly categorised into two types – propositional (formal) and non-propositional (personal) – and comes from three sources – tenacity, authority and a priori. Clinical knowledge can be seen as based on superstition, folklore, craft or science.
- Science is a body of knowledge organised in a systematic way based on observation, experiment and measurement.
- Evidence is information or data which supports or refutes beliefs in relation to a particular area of interest.
- Evidence on which to base nursing practice is best drawn from a variety of credible sources reflecting the multifaceted and complex needs of nursing. There are four types of evidence on which nurses can base their practice – research, clinical experience, service user/carer perspectives and local context.
- There are 'ready made' forms of evidence available, where best evidence has been collected and summarised, such as clinical guidelines and summaries.
- Appropriate, focused questions are the backbone of EBP. The PICO format is helpful in the development of questions related to effectiveness, PICo for those related to feasibility, meaning and appropriateness.

Further reading

Carper, B. (1978) 'Fundamental patterns of knowing in nursing', *Advances in Nursing Science*, 1: 13–23. For a full exploration of the nature of nursing knowledge.

Dawson, D. and Endacott, R. (2011) 'Implementing quality initiatives using bundled approach', *Intensive Critical Care Nursing*, 27: 117–120. Gives an overview of the development of care bundles.

Stillwell, S.B., Fineout-Overholt, E., Melnyk, B.M. and Williamson, K.M. (2010) 'Asking the clinical question: A key step in evidence-based practice', *American Journal of Nursing*, 110(3): 58–61. For further exploration of the use of PICO in question formation.

E-resources

Netting the Evidence: Google Search Engine: searches 107 sites associated with EBP. http://tinyurl.com/2poh3a

Trip Database: a search engine that identifies high quality evidence for use in clinical practice. www.tripdatabase.com

NHS Evidence: enables users to simultaneously search 150 data sources for resources such as clinical summaries, guidelines, research literature, British National Formulary. www.evidence.nhs.uk

Clinical Knowledge Summaries: provides concise summaries of evidence related to common primary care issues and gives recommendations for practice. www.cks.library.nhs.uk

3

Patients' Perspectives and Shared Decision Making

Learning Outcomes

By the end of the chapter you will be able to:

- discuss the issues related to patient involvement;
- consider appropriate ways of incorporating the patient's perspective into decision-making processes;
- develop and use appropriate resources to facilitate shared decision-making processes.

Introduction

The NHS Plan (DH, 2001a) set out a 10-year programme for improving the healthcare services in the UK. It identified three phases to this improvement: putting in place structures to ensure services were delivered appropriately; making the service more responsive to the needs of modern society; and promoting safe and clinically effective care which would enhance patient experience. Central to all these phases was the involvement of service users in the decisions made about their care. More recently, the White Paper *Equality and Excellence: Liberating the NHS* (DH, 2010) advocated **shared decision making** (SDM) and stated that 'no decision about me, without me' was to become the mantra of future care delivery. The NMC (2008) clearly outlines in the Code of Conduct the expectation that nurses will work collaboratively with patients, and Coulter and Collins (2011) have stated that health professionals are ethically obligated to discuss treatment options with patients and determine their individual preferences. As discussed in Chapter 1 the involvement of patients in decision making is essential to EBP and both government and professional bodies seem to see this as a key issue when considering the delivery of care.

Patient perspectives

There is a potential tension between EBP as a scientific approach to care – based on sound evidence – and the underlying health philosophy of care being patient-centred, requiring nursing in particular to respond holistically to the individual needs of patients. However Sidani et al. (2006) suggested the two approaches are complementary as both aim at ensuring that care is acceptable to the patient and delivered in the most effective way.

Patient preferences and experiences can be garnered in two ways – from individual patients or collations of multiple sources. There are a number of possible ways in which to gather a general understanding of collated patient preferences (see Box 3.1). These can give a general insight into how patients view certain aspects of care; what might impact on uptake of treatment and the continuation of treatment regimes; and the factors that lead to dissatisfaction. This information can also be useful when discussing options with individual patients as it can provide a background for discussions and exploring specific issues that may be of concern to individuals. It can also provide a source of information to include in your decision-making processes, by identifying possible issues you may need to take into consideration that individual patients have not identified.

Box 3.1   Collated patients' perspectives

- Research studies considering patient opinions.
- Local service user organisations (e.g. Help the Aged in the case of older people, MIND for mental health topics).
- National bodies (e.g. Long Term Conditions Alliance, Patients Association, Expert Patient Programme, Centre for Mental Health).
- Own institution's audits and service evaluation reports.

Activity

Select a topic of interest related to the delivery of care in your area of practice. Chose and locate two sources of information highlighted in Box 3.1 and identify potential patient perspectives in relation to that topic area.

As identified above, service user involvement is central to government policy. In 2003 the Department of Health document *Building on the Best: Choice, Responsiveness and Equity in the NHS* reported on a consultation of over 110,000 people and identified that people want to be involved in the decisions made about their health and healthcare. The type of experience patients want from the NHS was defined as:

- getting good treatment in a comfortable, caring and safe environment, delivered in a calm and reassuring way;
- having information to make choices, to feel confident and to feel in control;
- being talked to and listened to as an equal; being treated with honesty, respect and dignity.

These criteria appear to incorporate the essential elements of patient-centred care (see Box 3.2). Amongst the various commitments made by the government in this document is a pledge to 'ensure people have the right information, at the right time, with the support they need to use it so that this becomes central to how we care for people' (DH, 2003: 9). Yet there is strong evidence to suggest that patients continue to have little input into the decisions made about their treatment and care (see, for example, Davis et al., 2010).

Box 3.2   Characteristics of patient-centred care

- Recognising the patient as a unique individual with specific:

  - beliefs/values;
  - needs;
  - preferences;
  - experience;
  - concerns.

- Responding flexibly to the patient in the provision of care, ensuring it reflects his/her individual:

  - needs;
  - preference;
  - concerns.

Activity

Reflect on a recent experience in practice where changes have been made to a patient's care regime. How much involvement did the patient have in the decision processes? Could this be improved and if so how?

In 2012, the DH White Paper *Liberating the NHS: No Decision About Me, Without Me* stated that shared decision making (SDM) was to be the foundation to all healthcare pathways. Traditionally the model of care in the health setting has been what is termed 'paternalistic', where it is expected that patients will comply with the 'orders' of health professionals. Recent years have seen a move towards 'consumer involvement' both in government policy and service user movements. Three models of service user involvement have previously been proposed (see Table 3.1), the basic foundation of all three was to ensure that patients were included at various levels of decision-making processes (Barker and Rush, 2009).

Table 3.1 Models of user involvement

Model	Description
Consumerist	• Emerged in the late 1980s/early 1990s • Service users seen as customers and/or consumers of the health services • Emphasises increased choice
Democratic	• Appeared in mid-1990s • Sought to equal the balance of power between professionals and patients, by empowering service users • Advocated the involvement of service users in decision making
Stakeholder	• Grew out of the democratic approach in the late 1990s • Emphasises a partnership between all stakeholders – patients, professionals, government – to ensure all have equal influence on the development of services and delivery of care

However SDM, the approach now being advocated, is seen as somewhat different to the above as its focus is on decision making in relation to treatment preferences and on decision making being shared equally. SDM is seen to provide better health outcomes, better adherence to treatment regimes and higher levels of patient satisfaction (Singh et al., 2010). Therefore it would seem both clinically and cost effective to promote some form of partnership working between service users and health professionals. The concept of individual patient involvement requires health professionals to recognise the active role of patients in ensuring healthcare is safe, effective and meets their needs. Many service users expect to be involved in decisions related to their health treatment options and care, and 'bring different but equally important forms of expertise to the decision-making process' (Coulter and Collins, 2011: 2). The professionals' expertise lies in their knowledge of the disease processes and treatment options available; the patients bring their experience and understanding of the impact of the disease on their everyday lives and their personal preference, attitudes and values.

There are certain characteristics associated with SDM:

- the sharing of information between at least two individuals;
- all parties making and agreeing the decision;
- an ongoing partnership between the patient and the clinical team.

Best and Hagen (2010) proposed that the approach involves working collaboratively with patients by:

1 Listening to and exploring what a patient knows about their health problems and care
  needs.
2 Providing opportunities to express concerns and worries.
3 Discussing possible treatment options.
4 Providing appropriate information about these options.
5 Making sure information is understood.
6 Ensuring decisions reflect patient's wishes.
7 Offering regular opportunities to review decisions.

Involving patients in decision making assumes that they are motivated and have the
power and ability to be involved in decisions made about their healthcare. In reality
some patients want to be more involved than others. Hack et al. (1994) proposed
that five decision control positions (preferred level of involvement) were possible:

1 Active.
2 Active shared.
3 Collaborative.
4 Passive shared.
5 Passive.

In meta-analysis studies investigating the preferred level of involvement in decision
making of people with physical illnesses, Singh et al. (2010) found 26 per cent of
people preferred an active/active passive role; 49 per cent a collaborative role; and
25 per cent a passive role in healthcare decision-making processes. Adams et al.
(2007) undertook a similar small study of people with severe mental illness and found
64 per cent of participants expressed a preference for a collaborative approach in the
mental health setting. It would seem that the majority of patients, irrespective of the health
issue, prefer a collaborative approach to decision making. There is clearly a need to
check what level of involvement a patient wants in the decision-making process.

Activity

Consider your current areas of practice and identify patients who appear to want to be
involved in the decision process and those who do not. What might be the reasons for these
differences?

It is suggested that younger people and those people with higher educational levels
often want to take a more active role in decisions made about their care. However,
it is possible that a preference for an active role in healthcare decisions may be a

personality trait rather than a group-specific characteristic. Therefore it is important to check all patients' preferred level of involvement.

Involving patients in decision making is not without its problems. As Ervin and Pierangeli (2005) identified a person's level of self-confidence may impact on their willingness to participate in decision making. There is a potential for power struggles if the patient's preference runs counter to what professionals think is the most effective or feasible treatment or chooses an option that is thought to be detrimental to their well-being. Michaels et al. (2008) cautioned that tensions can arise if patients reject professionals' recommendations. Equally there may be difficulties in relation to a patient's perspectives and that of their family members, who, believing they have their loved ones' best interests at heart, advocate different approaches to treatment.

As identified earlier, not all patients want to be involved in decision-making processes. Whilst it is essential that they are provided with the appropriate information and informed consent is obtained before any care is delivered, it must be remembered that patients have the right to choose what level of involvement they wish to have (Crib and Entwistle, 2011). However the main challenges to SDM, according to Braddock (2010), centre on how to engage health professionals in this process – often clinicians make decisions without providing patients with information about options – and how to provide information for patients in a way that facilitates understanding of the issues under consideration.

Activity

Reflect on your own practice and identify if you actively involve patients in the decision-making process. If you do, how can you improve this? If you do not, consider how you can develop this aspect of your practice.

Involving patients in SDM

Accessing individual preferences from patients in your care and attempting to integrate patient preferences into clinical decisions is central to EBP. Sidani et al. (2006) identify this as a three-step process:

1 Identifying evidence on which to base care, accounting for alternative approaches to meet patient needs and preparing easy to understand descriptions of the evidence.
2 Informing patients of the possible options and identifying preferences.
3 Integrating patient preferences into the delivery of care.

As step 1 indicates it is essential that you have the full information regarding the proposed intervention(s) so you can ensure the patient has a complete understanding of the issues. Preparing a written description is often helpful as it can allow the patient to consider the information in a format that they can return to and take in at their own pace. (Appendix 2 provides a possible template for providing this information.)

Activity

Identify an aspect of care relevant to your own area. Prepare a description of that aspect of care using the template provided in Appendix 2.

In writing for patients you need to ensure that you provide something that is accessible to them. The 'writing in plain language' movement advocates that information should be provided in a clear and straightforward way. Cutts (2009: vi) defined this as 'writing and setting out of essential information in a way that gives a co-operative, motivated person a good chance of understanding it at first reading and in the same sense that the writer means it to be understood'. Box 3.3 identifies some of the basic things to consider when preparing written resources for patients. The Plain English Campaign site offers some resources which may be of use to you (see www.plainenglish. co.uk/).

Box 3.3   Writing in plain English

- Know your reader and aim at an average reader.
- Organise content – put most important information first or organise chronologically.
- Use headings to break up content.
- Use personal pronouns – you, I, we.
- Use an 'active voice' – 'you will experience' rather than the 'passive' voice.
- Short sentences (no more than 25 words) and short sections.
- Simple verb tense – 'you do' rather than 'you will do'.
- Simple structure – 'we manage care' rather than 'we are responsible for managing care'.
- Omit excess words – 'this is critical' rather than 'this is really critical'.
- Avoid jargon, foreign words, Latin or legal terms.
- Use lists or tables to simplify complex information.
- Get someone to proofread it for you.

The DISCERN initiative (Charnock, 1998) provided a tool to assess the quality of decision-making information provided to the patient. The intention was that this tool would be used by both patients and information providers and is a useful guide as to what should be included in patient information.

Activity

Visit the DISCERN website at www.discern.org.uk. Compare the information you provided in the previous activity with the DISCERN criteria and identify if there are aspects you could improve.

As involving patients in decision making has become a central tenet of care a number of initiatives have been launched and resources developed. One example of this is the MAGIC (Making Good Decisions in Collaboration) programme, funded by the Health Foundation (see www.health.org.uk/magic). This is aimed at 'embedding shared decision making in everyday practice' by developing ways of promoting and supporting patients making informed decisions in specific areas (i.e. general practice, obstetric units, breast cancer units, ear, nose and throat departments and urology). It is also aimed at changing the culture in healthcare to enable healthcare staff to involve service users in decision making.

One such initiative is the 'Ask 3 Questions campaign' (see www.ask3questions. co.uk). Here resources have been developed to encourage patients to ask:

1 What are my options?
2 What are the possible benefits and risks of these options?
3 How likely are the benefits and risks of each option?
   (Health Foundation, 2012)

Option grids have also been developed to help identify areas of discussion in relation to specific treatment options.

Activity

Visit the Ask 3 Questions website (www.ask3questions.co.uk) and review the information and resources provided. Consider if and how the resources could be used in your current area of practice.

Standardised patient decision aids

Standardised **patient decision aids** (PDAs) are available to help facilitate patient decision making. These tools are usually generated following clinical research and studies of patients' information needs and guide patients through the decision-making process (O'Connor et al., 2004). PDAs have been well researched in some areas (such as breast cancer treatment) and less so in others (such as the mental health context). Nevertheless there is a growing body of research round these

approaches. It is intended that they will be used when there is more than one possible option available in relation to a particular health issue. Each PDA presents the
various risks and benefits of each option in a clear and simple way, enabling the
patient to make an informed choice based on their own preferences and values.
Many include ways of clarifying individuals' values and take patients through the
decision process step-by-step.

PDAs come in many forms – leaflets, interactive software, workbooks – and are
intended to be used by health professionals and patients to inform their discussions rather
than replace them. They do, however, provide information in a format that patients can
consider at their own pace and in their own time, and then return to in the discussions of
options with health professionals. It is suggested that the PDAs do three things:

1   Provide an overview of the facts relating to the intervention option.
2   Help people to clarify their preferences and values.
3   Provide a means of communicating these to health professionals.

The Cochrane Review Team of Patient Decision Aids create and review decision aids;
a register of these can be found on the Collaboration's site (www.ohri.ca/decisionaids).

Activity

Visit the Decision Aids website and identify a tool relevant to your area of practice. Consider
whether the tool would be useful in helping you to gain an overview of a patient's preferences
and how you might use it.

Engaging patients in decision-making activities

Gaining a patient's perspective requires giving your full attention to the individual's
'narrative' – their story – and enabling them to freely express their beliefs, values and
concerns in a non-judgemental and supportive way. This requires you to have good
communication and interpersonal skills and the ability to build a trusting relationship
with the patient. It is not in the remit of this chapter to consider these issues in any
depth. However, Kitson (2002) suggests there are basic skills underpinning this activity:

- knowing what questions to ask;
- using active listening skills;
- having an awareness of the principles underpinning patient-centred care;
- putting the principles of patient-centred care into practice;
- being open to new ideas and alternative ways of thinking;
- making explicit links between different sources of knowledge, evidence and decision-
  making processes.

Activity

Choose one of Kitson's (2002) basic skills identified above. Undertake a SWOT analysis – see the template in Appendix 1 – in relation to your skills in this area. Then develop an action plan identifying how you will develop this aspect in order to enhance your EBP activities.

Consent and capacity

Legislation relating to consent, mental capacity and competency is central to patient involvement and decision making, and therefore must be considered when involving patients in SDM. The NMC (2008) emphasises that patients have the right to be involved in all aspects of decision making and that nurses have a duty to obtain consent before any care is given. It also stipulates that individuals have the right to accept or refuse treatment and their decisions should be respected and supported. However, the Mental Capacity Act (MCA) (DH, 2005a) may have implications for certain aspects of consent in specific circumstances, particularly where health issues may impact on capacity to consent to treatment or an individual has learning disabilities.

The MCA (DH, 2005a) allows for others to make decisions if the patient's capacity to do so is compromised through mental health issues, learning disabilities (intellectual disabilities), drink, drugs, pain, fear, or the effects of physical diseases. A person's capacity to consent may fluctuate, temporarily or permanently, or may relate to certain aspects of care – individuals may have the capacity to make certain decisions, but not others. However it must not be automatically assumed that people do not have the capacity to make decisions, the default position is always that 'a person is assumed to have capacity unless it is established that he lacks capacity' (DH, 2005a: section 1(2)).

The MCA also stipulates that someone must not be considered incapable until all possible ways of helping the person have been explored. It stresses that capacity should not be confused with the health professional's view of the reasonableness of a decision (i.e. that a particular choice is seen as unwise from a professional perspective). Where capacity is in doubt a full assessment must be carried out which considers the individual's ability to:

- understand information relevant to the decision;
- retain the information;
- weigh up information as part of the decision-making process;
- communicate effectively – verbally, sign language or muscle movement such as blinking.

The MCA clearly outlines the processes that must be in place before someone is considered not to have the capacity to be involved in decisions about their healthcare.

SDM in the mental health setting

The advent of the 'recovery' model in mental health, which emphasises the importance of incorporating service users' values and preferences in the delivery of care, would seem to indicate that the adoption of SDM is essential. The recovery model advocates the need to empower service users and promotes collaboration between professionals, the carers and the individual. SDM in mental health has been shown to improve adherence to treatment regimes and service user satisfaction (Drake et al., 2012) and research in this area is growing. However as Adams et al. (2007) identified, service users frequently feel they are not involved in decision-making processes and Deegan and Drake (2006) noted there is a need for more work in this area, calling for the development of PDAs specifically designed to support people with mental health problems.

There are specific barriers to SDM in mental health:

- the traditional use of a medical/disease focused treatment model;
- mental health professionals' legal and moral obligation to the service user and society to prevent harm to self and/or others;
- expectations of others – professional agencies and informal carers;
- service users' competence, insight and mental state.

Despite these issues, increasingly service users, their carers and mental health professionals are looking for ways to promote SDM.

The National Institute for Health and Clinical Excellence (2009) has advocated the use of '**advanced decisions**' in mental health settings, for people with schizophrenia to overcome issues related to competency to make decisions due to mental health problems. Such advanced decisions are legally binding under the MCA (2005a) if they are seen as valid (the individual had capacity to make the decision at the time and has not expressed a change in opinion) and applicable (the need for treatment has come into effect and the individual is incapable of making the decision at that time).

Sidley (2012) suggested that for people with complex and/or severe mental health problems it can help to shape future treatment and is likely to have a positive impact on therapeutic outcomes. Service users and care providers often have different perspectives as to what are priorities in care and what represents a good outcome. For example Deegan and Drake (2006) discussed the perspectives people with mental health problems may have in relation to medications – such as the side effects being worse than the illness experience; there is only a need to take medication when they are experiencing distress. Practitioners are said to be more concerned with the effectiveness of medications in reducing symptoms of mental illness and preventing relapses. They advocate that anything that facilitates communication and offers involvement is likely to have a positive effect on patient recovery and see advanced directives as part of the shared decision-making process.

Activity

Locate the following article: Sidley, G. (2012) 'Advanced decisions in secondary mental health services', *Nursing Standard* 26(21) 44–48. Review the process described to implement advanced decisions and consider, if not already in place, whether a similar approach could be used in your own area of practice.

SDM in child health

Including children in the decision-making process is particularly complex and often requires consideration of the child's developmental stage and parental responsibility. Griffith and Tengnah (2012) identified three developmental stages:

1 Tender years – where the child is considered not to have decision-making competency, therefore decisions are made by whoever has parental responsibility for the child.
2 Gillick competent – where a child under the age of 16 years is assessed in terms of their maturity (experiences and ability to manage influences such as peer pressure) and intelligence (understanding and ability to weigh up the various benefits and risks and long-term impact of decisions). The more serious the decision, the greater the level of competency required.
3 Young persons – where 16- and 17-year-old individuals are allowed to consent and participate in decisions as if they were at the age of consent.

It is expected that children will be involved in the decision-making process at the level appropriate for their age, ability and experience (Coyne et al., 2011). Children with long-term illnesses are felt to have a high level of competence in making decisions. It is suggested that children feel more valued and less anxious when involved in decision processes and it is expected that health professionals are at least aware of and include children's views in making decisions about their care (Baston, 2008). Providing children with age-appropriate information – for example using play or dolls – enables them to cope better with their illness. However, as decision making involves three parties (child, parents and health professional) it can be particularly problematic.

Where parents are involved in decision making it has been found that the level of desired involvement can range from 'none' where this is seen as the nurse/doctor's role, to providing comfort, to acting as the child's advocate and having primary responsibility for making decisions (Franck et al., 2012). These seem to reflect the positions adopted by patients in terms of their preferred level of involvement in decision making.

Moore and Kirk (2010) identified a number of the factors that can enhance children's participation in decision making, an overview of these is provided in Box 3.4.

> ## Box 3.4   Enhancement of child involvement in decision making
>
> - Presence of parent.
> - Parents' approval of child's participation.
> - Parents with a good standard of education.
> - Child has a good understanding and knowledge about their condition.
> - Child has the ability to access information about their illness.
> - Age and maturity of child.
> - Experienced healthcare professionals.

Activity

Consider your own area of practice and identify what is available to facilitate children's involvement in decision making about their care. How could this be improved?

SDM in the learning disabilities setting

Valuing People: A New Strategy for the 21st Century (DH, 2001b) was the first White Paper for 30 years which specifically addressed the care of people with learning disabilities (LD). It had four central themes which would seem to reflect the SDM ethos:

1   Principles of choice.
2   Independence.
3   Rights.
4   Inclusion.

However various reports (such as *Healthcare for All: Report of the Independent Inquiry into Access to Healthcare for People with Learning Disabilities* [DH, 2008]) have demonstrated that people with learning disabilities continue to experience inequalities in the quality of care they receive. Most damning was the report *Death by Indifference* (Mencap, 2007), which described the deaths of six people with LD while receiving care in the NHS and attributed this to institutional discrimination against people with LD and a belief that they are not capable of being involved in decisions about their care.

Valuing People Now (DH, 2007b) identified the need for people with LD to have greater choice and control over their lives and support to develop person-centred plans. However it has also been shown that many healthcare professionals lack confidence in working with this group of people and limited understanding of their needs (Barr and Sowney, 2007).

There are a number of ways that people with learning disabilities can be involved in decision making such as:

- Gathering information from family/carers and friends with regard to the ways that the person communicates/responds to specific situations and undertakes daily activities.
- Developing individual support packages. This may mean providing information in picture form, using videos or using symbols.
- Identifying ways to facilitate meaningful communication such 'Intensive Interaction' (Nind and Hewitt, 2006). See www.intensiveinteraction.co.uk for further information.
- Providing accessible information. (See www.learningdisabilities.org.uk/publications/176171/ for an example of the types of information.)

Recent government policy (DH, 2007b) advocated the development of 'Circles of Support' as a way of supporting people with complex or severe LD in making decisions about care. These are 'a group of people who meet together on a regular basis to help somebody achieve their personal goals' (www.circlesnetwork.org.uk, 2012). Many people with learning disabilities will have an identified circle of support and it is essential that these people are involved in care decisions.

Activity

Consider your own area of practice and identify what is available to facilitate the involvement of people with learning disabilities in decision making about their care. How could this be improved?

EBP Activity

Ferguson and Day (2007) identified that novice nurses have difficulty in identifying patient preferences and values. Complete a SWOT analysis (refer to Appendix 1) and identify your future learning needs in this area.

Summary

- Involving service users in the decisions is central to EBP, affecting adherence to treatment and patient satisfaction.
- Patient preferences and experiences can be gleaned in two ways – from individual patients or collations of multiple sources.

(Continued)

(Continued)

- Patients may have different preferred levels of involvement. There is a need to check what level of involvement a patient wants in the decision-making process.
- The majority of patients, irrespective of the health issue, prefer a collaborative approach to decision making.
- There is a need to provide information for patients in a way that facilitates understanding of the issues under consideration.
- Standardised patient decision aids (PDAs) are available to help facilitate patient decision making.
- The Mental Capacity Act (DH, 2005a) allows for others to make decisions, only if the patient's capacity to do so is compromised

Further reading

Coulter, A. and Collins, A. (2011) *Making Shared Decision-Making a Reality: No Decision About Me, Without Me*. London: The Kings Fund; www.kingsfund.org.uk/publications/nhs_decisionmaking.html. Provides a good overview of shared decision making, approaches and methods of developing this in your own area of practice.

E-resources

NHS National Prescribing Centre: has a series of short videos related to EBP and decision making, including shared decision making and decision aids. www.npc.nhs.uk/evidence/making_decisions_better/making_decisions_better.php

Cochrane Collaboration of Patient Decision Aids (Ottawa Health Research Institute): provides a collection of patient decision aids. www.ohri.ca/decisionaid

Decision Aids Collection: provides links to a range of decision-making tools. www.thedecisionaidcollection.nl

MAGIC (Making Good Decisions in Collaboration): programme funded by the Health Foundation www.health.org.uk/magic

4

Clinical Judgement and Decision Making

Learning Outcomes

By the end of the chapter you will be able to:

- describe the nature of clinical judgement and decision making;
- identify the processes involved in clinical judgement and decision making;
- identify and use appropriate decision-making frameworks.

Introduction

Portney (2004) suggested that EBP should more correctly be called evidence-based decision making, as it requires practitioners to draw on a range of information and make a decision as to what is actually required. Melnyk and Fineout-Overholt (2005) have stated it is useful to think of EBP as requiring you to be involved in two essential activities – critically appraising evidence (discussed in Chapter 6) and using clinical judgement to consider how applicable the evidence is to your own area of practice.

It has been identified that prior to the advent of EBP most health professionals based clinical decision making on 'their vast educational knowledge coupled with intelligent guesswork, hunches and experience' (Pape, 2003: 155). Reliance on such approaches is no longer seen as appropriate. Clinical judgement and decision making are identified as central to clinical competence. Nursing not only involves knowing the how and why of delivering a certain type of care but also the ability to give sound rationales and justifications for clinical judgements and decisions taken. The NMC (2010) has now made decision making one of the four competency domains which must be acquired before registration, emphasising its importance in delivering professional care.

However decision making is not a straightforward activity. The increasing complexity of the care needs of individuals, care interventions and care delivery settings requires finely honed clinical judgement skills to ensure clinical decision making is of

the highest standard. Lamb and Sevdalis (2011) have identified that clinical judgement and decision-making skills take practitioners beyond purely technical or
knowledge-based skills, proposing these to be 'key non-technical' skills essential for
the safe delivery of care. Therefore these concepts will be explored here and the relationship between scientific knowledge and practice experience debated.

What is clinical judgement?

As identified above clinical judgement is an essential skill for all health professionals and
one that separates them from undertaking a purely technical role. Various terms are used
in relation to this activity (clinical reasoning, problem solving, critical thinking) but all are
related to the ability to consider the various issues at hand, make a judgement in relation
to the impact of the various elements and come up with a decision as to what appropriate
action to take. Levett-Jones et al. (2010) suggested there are five 'rights' in relation to this
concept – right cues, right patient, right action, right time for the right reason.

Decisions will have implications for patient outcomes and as such must deserve serious
consideration. No decision should ever be made without an accompanying judgement as
to the appropriateness of that decision. Tanner (2006: 204) defined clinical judgement as
'an interpretation or conclusion about a patient's needs ... and/or the decision to take
action' and suggests that there are various factors that impact on this process:

- nurses' experiences and perspectives/values – a 'knowing what to do' (these have a greater
  impact on clinical judgement than scientific evidence);
- a knowledge of the patient and their preferences – 'knowing the patient';
- the context and culture of the care environment – 'knowing their own environment where
  specific care will be delivered'.

There is a need to consider how the evidence relates to your practice context – is it
transferable; are there identifiable risks and/or benefits to using the evidence in your area
of practice? There also needs to be an evaluation of the options with an acceptance that
decisions made may vary from patient to patient in the same situations. For example
research evidence may suggest a certain course of action is appropriate in women aged
between 50 and 60 with leg ulcers or that a particular drug is the treatment of choice
for depression in adolescents. However in reality such interventions may not be appropriate for particular individuals whilst for others these are the treatment of choice.

Activity

Reflect on a recent practice experience where a particular intervention appeared more appropriate for some patients than others. What factors impacted on the suitability of specific
interventions for different individuals?

It is proposed that practitioners consider evidence in terms of its relevance and weight, however this is an individual assessment so what might be considered relevant and given greater weight by one clinician may not be considered in the same way by another (Lasater, 2011). In any two clinical situations the context and individual nurse's experience/knowledge will impact on the judgements and decisions made. All clinical judgements have ethical considerations, with the health professional weighing up the potential benefits and risks involved in any decision made. Frequently there are a number of options available, each of which carries its own risks and benefits. This adds another dimension to the decision-making process and often it is the patient's preferences that indicate which is the best choice (see Chapter 3). Therefore reflection is central to clinical judgement as it requires health professionals to consider and make links between the evidence, their own knowledge, skills and experience and that of other team members as well as patient preferences, beliefs and values. However for this to be effective in aiding clinical judgement it must be undertaken in a clear and structured way rather than simply 'thinking about' the issues. Reflection is explored further in Chapter 11, however it is useful to consider the issues specific to clinical decision making here.

It has been identified that appropriate reflection and particularly reflective writing encourage the transfer of knowledge from one situation to another and help in knowledge transformation – consideration of the relevance current experiences may have for future activities (Nielsen et al., 2007). It is also proposed that this promotes the development of critical thinking – a central component of clinical judgement. Nielsen et al. (2007) have provided a guide for reflection aimed at developing clinical judgement skills.

Activity

Locate the following article: Nielsen, A., Stragnell, S. and Jester, P. (2007) 'Guide for reflection using the Clinical Judgement Model', *Journal of Nursing Education*, 46(11): 513–516. Using Nielsen et al.'s guide, reflect on a recent incident from your own area of practice.

The reasoning processes used in clinical judgement tend to be described as involving either analytical or intuitive activities (Tanner, 2006). The former involves the breaking down of a problem into its constituent parts, considering these, and weighing up the alternative approaches available in solving the problem. Usually this involves the processing of scientific data. Intuitive processes are seen as drawing on inherent knowledge, skills and experiences to find the answer to the problem. These two options are often seen as the opposite poles of a continuum. However, the idea of a 'cognitive continuum' is possibly more helpful in understanding the processes involved as these two activities are not 'mutually exclusive' (Standing, 2008: 127). Different approaches can be used in different situations depending on the complexity, ambiguity and presentation of the issue and both may be necessary when dealing with uncertain situations. The more complex, familiar or urgent the issue the more likely you are to rely on intuition. Any combination of these three elements will result in the use of differing levels of analysis and/or intuition.

Standing (2008) provided a cognitive continuum of clinical judgement in nursing based on identifying nine cognitive modes used by nurses in practice (see Table 4.1). No one mode is seen as more important than another, these simply reflected the types of knowledge drawn on in the clinical judgement and decision-making processes of nurses and the sort of activities nurses are likely to engage in. The intuitive mode is seen most frequently in face-to-face encounters with patients, whereas the experimental research mode is related to establishing effectiveness of intervention and is more distant from day-to-day care activities.

Table 4.1   Cognitive mode of nursing practice

Judgement process	Description
Intuitive	Drawing on tacit knowledge and arriving at a judgement without being aware of the process by which it was reached. Usually occurs in face-to-face care delivery situation.
Reflective	Incorporates both reflection in and on care delivery actions.
Patient and peer assisted	Encompasses seeking patient preferences and/or the expertise of other healthcare professionals.
System assisted	Involves the use of guidelines, problem-solving frameworks and decision aids.
Critical review of evidence (experience and research)	Identification of relevant information and application of this to the current situation.
Action research and audit	Gathering information through implementing and evaluating changes to care delivery systems.
Qualitative research	Seeking to understand the patient's experience and inform future practice by undertaking qualitative research.
Survey research	Answering questions related to future care delivery by collecting data via surveys.
Experimental research	Testing the effectiveness of intervention through the use of experimental research designs such as RCTs.

Activity

Consider the last clinical decision you made. How did you arrive at the decision? Were you aware of analysing the various aspects of the issue or was it reached more intuitively?

It has been proposed that an over-reliance on intuition may give rise to problems associated with bias – an under- or over-estimation of the importance of certain factors or information. Bias in the form of stereotyping, prejudice or selective memory can influence how you perceive and respond to information and individual patients. Equally, basing judgements and decision purely on your own experience and personal knowledge result in important research evidence being ignored or undervalued. Hammond (2007) identified that where analytical approaches to decision making are used errors occur infrequently but when they do they are often on a large scale; whereas errors resulting from intuition-based approaches occur frequently but tend to be small in nature. It is therefore essential that as a nurse you can defend judgements and justify how you reached these and the decisions made.

What is clinical decision making?

Thompson and Stapley (2011) proposed that clinical judgement and clinical decision making are closely linked but separate concepts. The former is about an evaluation of a situation, and the latter is concerned with whether or not to take action and what type of action to take if necessary. For example you might consider that a particular patient's diet is poor (judgement) and choose to provide them with an education package related to healthy eating (decision). Benner et al. (1996: 2) suggested that clinical judgement relates to 'the ways in which nurses come to understand the problems, issues, or concerns of clients/patients, to attend to salient information and to respond in concerned and involved ways'. In this way decision making is seen as an interaction between three things – the patient's preferences (discussed in Chapter 3); the evidence available on which to base practice; and the clinical judgement of the nurse involved based on personal experience and knowledge. These three components come together to produce a clinical decision as to what action should be taken – see Figure 4.1.

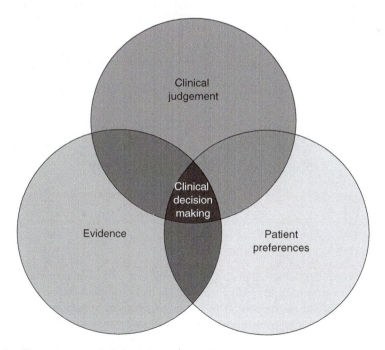

Figure 4.1 Components of clinical decision making

Poor decision making in nursing usually happens when nurses use the wrong type of information to inform their decisions or place too much emphasis on a particular form of information (Dowding and Thompson, 2004). Therefore it is crucial to ensure that when making decisions the appropriate sources of information are accessed. When studying decision making in nurses, Rycroft-Malone et al. (2009) found that nurses used a range of strategies, drawing on informal protocols – local ways of working – interactions with co-workers and patients, instinct and formal protocols. However the primary approach used was interactions with others: here nurses discussed decisions made with colleagues and preferred to approach more senior colleagues for information rather than turning to protocols. Protocol-based care has generally been advocated as helping health professionals reach the 'best' decision in relation to the situation they seek to facilitate. It is said these simplify and aid decision making, promoting standardised practice based on best available evidence in the form of care pathways, guidelines and/or algorithms. Rycroft-Malone et al. (2009) found that less experienced staff tended to use protocols more frequently but as individuals become more experienced there was a tendency to rely on memory and past experiences Although nurses recognised that protocols should be used more frequently, time constraints were said to reduce ability to refer to these. Protocols were often referred to after delivering care to see if decisions made fell within stated guidelines. Nurses expressed a belief that protocols encouraged standardisation, which it was felt did not necessarily equate to best practice as it was seen as being impersonal and therefore challenged individualisation of care.

There are many different types of clinical decisions which nurses are called upon to make. Thompson et al. (2004) identified 11 different forms of decisions made in everyday practice (see Box 4.1).

Box 4.1   Forms of decisions made in practice

Intervention	Targeting	Timing	Prevention
Referral	Communication	Assessment	Diagnosis
Information	Experience	Service delivery	

Activity

Reflect on one recent day in clinical practice and consider if, when and how you were involved in the 11 types of decisions identified in Table 4.2. Identify how these decisions were made and whether you felt you had the appropriate evidence on which to base those decisions.

There are various conceptual models available to explain the factors involved in making a clinical decision. Tanner (2006) proposed that it is a four-stage process involving noticing, interpreting, responding and reflecting. Lasater (2006) identifies that each of these stages has specific components:

1 Noticing – observing, noticing change and collecting information.
2 Interpreting – making sense of the information and prioritising.
3 Responding – planning intervention, using clear communication and appropriate skills.
4 Reflecting – evaluating the incident and looking for ways to improve performance.

Standing (2011) suggested that clinical decision-making skills have 10 facets (see Box 4.2).

Box 4.2   Clinical decision-making skills

Collaboration   Experience and intuition   Confidence
Systematic   Prioritising   Observation
Standardisation   Reflectivity   Ethical sensitivity
Accountability

Activity

Identify one patient whose care you were recently involved with. Consider each of Standing's decision-making skills and identify whether or not you used these in making care delivery decisions.

In making a clinical decision, it is proposed that a nurse's judgement is helped if the most up-to-date evidence is available and the needs of the service user are clearly identified. However, simply providing nurses with appropriate evidence will not in itself enhance the decision-making processes. Thompson (2003) put forward the notion of 'clinical uncertainty' in relation to decision making, the idea that the practice of nursing takes place in the face of ever-changing demands. A patient's needs and status will change over time, thus resulting in complex and often competing demands.

If decision making is to be effective then health professionals need to be aware of such changes and factor them into any decisions to be made. Therefore it is necessary to consider the implications of a decision over time, what Melnyk and Fineout-Overholt (2005) describe as 'clinical forethought'. This has four components – future think, forethought about specific populations, anticipation of risks and the unexpected (see Table 4.2 for an overview). Issues that may have an impact on, and implications for, care delivery should be identified and considered. Clinical judgement is used in managing these uncertainties and arriving at a decision as to how to proceed – many see this as the 'art' of nursing – and is central to clinical expertise.

Table 4.2   Clinical forethought

Type	Description
Future think	<ul><li>Considering the immediate future and anticipating issues that might arise</li><li>Identifying immediate resources needed</li><li>Considering future responses</li><li>Evaluating judgement and making adjustments as necessary</li></ul>
Specific patients	<ul><li>Considering general trends in patient experiences and responses to intervention</li><li>Identifying local resources available to deal with potential issues</li></ul>
Risks	<ul><li>Anticipating particular issues that may impact on a specific individual – such as anxiety, distress</li></ul>
The unexpected	<ul><li>Expecting the unexpected</li><li>Anticipating the need to respond to new situations and resources – yours and organisational – if difficulties arise</li></ul>

Activity

Imagine you are about to administer a new form of medication to a patient for the first time. What 'clinical forethought' issues can you identify?

As identified above, nurses' personal knowledge and experience have the greatest impact on these decision-making activities, moulding how the nurse interprets the situation and deals with the uncertainties. The greater your knowledge/experience, the larger the number of perspectives and possibilities you are likely to identify. As discussed in Chapter 2, Benner (1984) proposed that the 'expert' nurse draws on knowledge in an intuitive way and reaches conclusions without being able to verbalise the process by which those decisions were reached (see Chapter 2 in relation to tacit knowledge). However Fitzpatrick (2007) suggested an expert nurse in relation to EBP needs to be able to make clear and reasoned links between theory and practice with the ability to integrate patient perspectives into this 'mix'.

Nursing expertise is defined by Titchen and Higgs (2001: 274) as the 'professional artistry and practice wisdom inherent in professional practice'. Clinical expertise is viewed by Manley et al. (2005) as having a number of components (see Box 4.2). The development of these aspects of clinical expertise are said to be linked to 'enabling factors' – the ability to reflect; to organise practice giving consideration to overarching influences; to work autonomously; to develop good interpersonal relationships; and to promote respect.

Box 4.3 Nursing expertise

1 Holistic practice knowledge – integrating various forms of knowledge, academic and experiential, into their delivery of care.
2 Knowing the patient – respecting the patient's views/perspectives, encouraging patient decision making and promoting independence.
3 Moral agency promoting respect, dignity and self-efficacy in others whilst maintaining own professional integrity.
4 Saliency – observing and picking up on cues from patients, recognising the needs of patients and others.
5 Skilled know-how – problem solving, responding to changing environment of care and adapting to needs as appropriate.
6 Change catalyst – promoting appropriate change.
7 Risk taker – weighing the risks and taking appropriate decisions, to achieve best patient outcomes.

Approaches to decision making

There are a number of frameworks that can be used to help with decision making. Below are just two that you may find helpful.

Facione (2007) offered a six-step approach to effective thinking and problem solving which he proposed involves five 'whats' and a 'why':

1 What is the question facing you?
2 What are the circumstances that surround the problem?
3 What are the most reasonable top three or four options?
4 What is the best course of action?

5   Why are you choosing this particular option?
6   What did you miss?

Activity

Consider an area of concern in your area of practice. Using Facione's framework identify how best to address the issues of concern.

Hoffman et al. (2010) proposed a clinical reasoning cycle, based on research concerning expert nurses' thought and decision-making processes. It was suggested that this cycle can be used to promote the development of practice-specific knowledge and clinical reasoning skills in students and novice practitioners. There are eight steps in the cycle:

1   Describe the patient and the context of their care situation.
2   Consider all the information currently available (notes, charts, history) and gather any further information needed. Apply the theoretical knowledge you already have to the patient's illness/presentation and the situation.
3   Review all the data you have to get a full picture of the patient and their context. Identify what is and is not relevant, and any patterns and relationships between the various pieces of information. Compare the current situation to your past experiences and suggest possible outcomes.
4   Evaluate the information to clarify the nature of the problem to be addressed.
5   Set your goals and time frame within which these will be achieved.
6   Implement your plan of action.
7   Evaluate outcomes.
8   Reflect on the experience and identify learning needs.

Activity

When in your own area of practice use Hoffman et al.'s framework in relation to a specific patient problem.

EBP calls for a more analytical approach to making clinical decisions, and it is anticipated there will be a conscious weighing up of the options and consideration of the various issues. The McMaster's EBM group caution against the use of clinical experience and intuition in the absence of evidence based on systematic observation in making clinical judgements (Eraut, 2000). However you should not underestimate how much interpretation may be needed in deciding how evidence should be used – EBP cannot always provide concrete evidence on which to base practice. A possible model for this process is given in Figure 4.2.

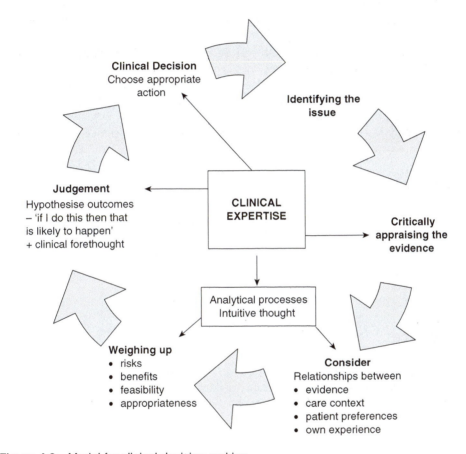

Figure 4.2 Model for clinical decision making

EBP Activity

Ferguson and Day (2007) proposed that novice nurses lack confidence in their own clinical judgement and decision-making processes. Complete a SWOT analysis (see Appendix 1) in relation to your own skills in this area and identify your future learning needs.

Summary

- The complexity of the care requires finely honed clinical judgement skills to ensure clinical decision making is of the highest standard.
- Nurses' experiences and perspectives/values have a greater impact on their clinical judgement than scientific evidence.
- Clinical judgement and clinical decision making are closely linked but separate concepts.
- Involvement of service users in the decisions and sound clinical decision making are central to EBP.
- Clinical judgement is seen as the 'art' of nursing and central to clinical expertise, and involves the weighing up of options and reaching a decision as to appropriate action.
- Both analytical process and intuitive thinking are central to clinical judgement.

Further reading

Standing, M. (2011) *Clinical Judgement and Decision Making for Nursing Students*. Exeter: Learning Matters. Provides an in-depth exploration of decision-making processes.

Thompson, C. and Dowding, D. (2009) *Essential Decision Making and Clinical Judgement for Nurses*. Amsterdam: Elsevier. Provides an in-depth exploration of issues related to clinical judgement and decision making.

E-resources

NHS National Prescribing Centre: has a series of short videos related to EBP and decision making, including individual decision making. www.npc.nhs.uk/evidence/making_decisions_better/making_decisions_better.php

5

Finding the Evidence

Learning Outcomes

By the end of the chapter you will be able to:

- identify how to search for relevant literature;
- choose appropriate databases to use in searching for evidence;
- understand the use of MeSH/subject headings, keyword, truncation and wildcards in searching for evidence.

Introduction

Searching for evidence can be both bewildering and complex, as Bartelt et al. (2011) discovered, health professionals often identify 'lack of search skills' – knowing how to find the evidence – as a personal barrier to implementing EBP. However it is an important skill to develop and as Greenhalgh (2006) has already pointed out you may be rigorous in critically appraising the evidence but if you are considering the wrong paper then this is a waste of your time and effort. Most forms of evidence are now available electronically so an important part of finding the evidence is being able to navigate your way through the various electronic systems involved. This chapter will introduce you to some of the key aspects related to finding the right evidence.

Where is the evidence?

Evidence is often viewed as being published materials only, but it can take many forms. The value and credibility of each type has to be considered when trying to establish if it is going to be useful to you. Books are often the first point of access for many people and remain a useful source of background information. However, these do not always provide the most up-to-date evidence. Journals can provide a range of articles, from research papers to discussion pieces. Research studies, as we have already seen, are generally viewed as being important forms of evidence.

Discussion and commentary papers can also be equally important when considering concepts and theories that are central to a profession's knowledge base or where little is known about a topic. In addition government and policy documents can prove a valuable source of information.

Another important source of evidence is what is known as **grey literature**. This is literature which has not been formally published, but nevertheless may include useful information. Usually grey literature is said to include:

- theses and/or dissertations – projects undertaken as part of a course of study for various levels of degree (masters and doctorates);
- conference proceedings which provide information not available in print;
- in-house publications – leaflets, newsletters, pamphlets.

What resources are available to help with EBP

With the explosion of information and knowledge available on which to base practice, busy practitioners can find themselves overwhelmed, and almost drowning in a sea of evidence. There is also an issue of ensuring that you find the best evidence in relation to your area of interest – not all literature is good evidence and you need to learn to distinguish between what is appropriate and what is not. DiCenso et al. (2009) identified six types of resources available to help practitioners find appropriate evidence to use when making decisions about care delivery, which are all pre-assessed resources having undergone filtering processes to ensure that only high quality studies are included. These are regularly updated and provide practitioners with easily accessed sources of information to ensure the evidence is current. The advantage of these pre-assessed resources is that they save practitioners time as the normal **critical appraisal** processes required in EBP have already been completed. DiCenso et al. arranged these in a hierarchy, with systems providing the highest and most useful form of information on which to base EBP:

1 Systems.
2 Summaries.
3 Synopses of syntheses.
4 Syntheses.
5 Synopses of single studies.
6 Critically appraised individual studies.

Systems are described as clinical decision support systems which can integrate and summarise all available, appropriate evidence related to a particular clinical issue and when linked to a specified patient's circumstances propose appropriate action (such as Clinical Evidence – www.clinicalevidence.bmj.com).

Summaries provide a summary of best practice, however these are different from textbooks in that they require a systematic approach to identifying, grading and summarising data and are date stamped with an updating schedule included. These usually take the form of best evidence summaries produced, for instance, by NICE, Joanna Briggs Best Practice Guidelines or the National Guidelines Clearinghouse.

Synopses of syntheses are concise descriptions of systematic reviews such as those produced by the Database of Abstracts of Reviews of Effects (DARE). Syntheses in the form of systematic reviews provide rigorous reviews of evidence relating to specific areas of interest, and are also advocated as good sources of information. These can be found in the Cochrane and Joanna Briggs Institute libraries.

Synopses of studies are summaries of individual studies, providing sufficient detail to make decisions as to whether something is relevant to your area of practice and could be incorporated into clinical actions. These can be seen in the form of abstracts that appear in the journal *Evidence-Based Nursing*. DiCenso et al. (2009) proposed that if evidence is not available in one of the above five resources there are electronic sites where single articles, deemed to meet specified standards, are made available, such as Evidence Updates.

It is proposed that health professions should start their search for evidence at the highest level of the hierarchy – systems – and if information is not available to work their way down the hierarchy (Bejaimal et al., 2012). This is seen as being the most effective approach to retrieving evidence as it stops you 'having to re-invent the wheel' as it were. If the information is already summarised and available it is a waste of your time and effort to go through the process again. If your area of interest is not covered by any of the six pre-assessed resources then your ultimate sources will be original studies and often the starting point for EBP. However you need to have the skills and tools to enable you to find and use these resources.

Searching

Searching for evidence is a skill that takes time and practice to develop and it is important that you get all the help you can. Many of the tools discussed below will have tutorials that talk you through the steps you need to take to make best use of the resources. It is well worth spending some time working through these. I would also advise that you make friends with your local librarian, who can help you develop the skills you need. Also book a training session with the librarian, your personal tutor or the information technologist for your school or health organisation to work through the basics of navigating the electronic systems. It will be time well spent and save you a great deal of effort and frustration later when you are searching for evidence to support your practice.

The first step in searching for evidence is deciding what it is you want to find. As discussed in Chapter 2 you need to decide what your focus is and identify a question using the PICO/PICo format. The terms you have identified in PICO will help you narrow down what you are actually looking for and can then form the basis of the terms you will use to search for appropriate evidence. In searching there is a need to consider:

- synonyms – words that share the same meaning (e.g. cancer and neoplasm);
- acronyms/abbreviations – where phrases have been shortened to a set of letters (e.g. CBT – cognitive behavioural therapy);
- alternative spellings (e.g. paediatrics and pediatrics);
- alternative terms (e.g. learning disabilities and learning disorders).

Activity

Identify an area you would like to know more about and generate a PICO/PICo question using the form in Appendix 3. Look at the words or phrases you have identified and consider what other words may be associated with them.

You may have come up with a long list or just a few phrases. Whichever is the case, these are what are known as your free text words/phrases. These are the words/phrases you can use to search for the evidence you need.

Manual searching

Your local library will have a range of resources that you can use to find the information needed. Most libraries have an electronic database of the books, journals and other resources available to its members. Using the words you have generated should help you to locate the information you want. Do not underestimate the resources the libraries have available, the most valuable being the librarians themselves – they are a key resource in finding the information you need.

Electronic searching

Today most people search electronic databases to ensure that they have the most up-to-date information and to increase their awareness of what is actually available on a given topic. Whilst libraries are often the first port of call, the physical resources within them are limited and there is often a need to look more widely.

Search engines

Search engines are designed to search for information on the World Wide Web. Google is the most popular and well-known search engine and is a useful tool.

However it is not sufficiently focused to meet all your needs when looking for evidence on which to base your practice and at the time of writing this book typing in the term 'learning disability' produced 65,600,000 results. It is essential that you do not rely on general search engines such as Google and that you instead familiarise yourself with and use those that are specifically aimed at the healthcare professions. A particular useful site is PubMed, which offers open access to MEDLINE listings and has a 'clinical queries' option. Here EBP filters are used to access relevant articles quickly. See Box 5.1 for examples of commonly used search engines.

Box 5.1   Commonly used search engines

Google and Google Scholar: provide access to electronic journal and textbooks.

Knowledge Finder: www.kfinder.com/newweb/

Turning Research into Practice (TRIP): a search engine for EBM. www.tripdatabase.com/

SUMSearch: searches various databases including MEDLINE, the National Guideline Clearing House and DARE. http://sumsearch.org

NHS Evidence: a search engine finding information relevant to health and social care from 150 different sources. www.evidence.nhs.uk/

PubMed: provides free web access to over 16 million citations from 5000 plus journals via MEDLINE and the US National Library of Medicine. http://pubmed.gov

---

Activity

Choose and locate one of the search engines identified in Box 5.1 (not Google). Type in the 'search box' one of the text words generated in the earlier activity. How many 'hits' are identified? Consider whether the results are sufficiently focused to meet your needs in searching for evidence.

Gateway sites

A **gateway site** will provide access to resources, databases and publications associated with a specific topic area. Some of these are free, others require a password. There are a growing number that are specific to healthcare professions. Box 5.2 outlines some of the most commonly used.

Box 5.2   Gateway sites

NHS Direct: another NHS site which provides various resources relevant to EBP. www.nhsdirect.nhs.uk

Centre for Reviews and Dissemination: conducts commissioned systematic reviews and provides access to the DARE and NHSEED databases. www.york.ac.uk/inst/crd

Netting the Evidence Google Search Engine: – searches 107 sites associated with EBP. http://tinyurl.com/2poh3a

RCN (Royal College of Nursing): – has it's own database accessible to members only, providing access to the British Nurse Index (and access to certain full text articles via CINAHL and MEDLINE. www.rcn.org.uk/development/library

Activity

Repeat the previous activity using one of the gateway sites identified in Box 5.2. Compare the results and consider the differences between the two sets of results.

Databases

Databases are a central point where details relating to certain types of information are gathered together. The ones that are of interest here are those related to the healthcare professions, and the most well known are listed in Box 5.3. The ones most commonly used by nurses are CINAHL (Cumulative Index to Nursing and Allied Health Literature) and MEDLINE. CINAHL is considered to be one of the most comprehensive databases for nurses and allied health professions. It has over 2.2 million records from 3000 plus journals, dating back to 1982 and covers all English-language journals. It also indexes some books, book chapters and nursing dissertations. There are various versions of CINAHL, from the original database to CINAHL Full Text plus. Access is through subscription only. So it will depend what your local provider subscribes to as to what is available to you.

MEDLINE is produced by the United States National Library of Medicine and carries over 21 million citations from over 5500 journals, with records going back to 1966. Although the majority of journals indexed are medical it also indexes a number of nursing journals. There are various online versions of MEDLINE and as mentioned above it can be freely accessed using PubMed.

There are a number of information service providers, through which education and health communities can access a range of data resources and support services from one platform. The most commonly used is Ovid, part of Wolters Kluwer

Health. The way data are accessed from databases and the methods of searching will be different depending on the provider's search engine. Therefore the easiest way to learn how to search the databases available to you is by asking your local librarian for a lesson or working through the online tutorials

---

Box 5.3   Commonly used bibliographic databases

CINAHL (Cumulative Index to Nursing and Allied Health Literature): literature relating to nursing and allied health professions from over 2928 journals, dating back to 1982. In looking for evidence this is a key source of information and often the place most nurses start.

MEDLINE: primary source for biomedical data from 1966 to the present. Complied by the US National Library of Medicine.

AMED: allied and complementary medicine database. Includes citations from 596 journals related to allied health professions, complementary medicine and palliative care.

EMBASE – Excerpta Medica Online: similar to MEDLINE but having a focus on drugs and pharmacology.

PsychINFO: has a database of publications which reaches back to the late 19th century related to psychology and allied fields such as mental health nursing and psychiatry.

Cochrane Database of Systematic Reviews: regularly updated systematic reviews.

BNI (British Nurse Index): database of over 260 nursing, midwifery and allied professions journals from 1994 to the present.

DARE (Database of Abstracts of Reviews of Effect): contains over 5000 appraisals of systematic reviews not found in the Cochrane database.

SCOPUS: contains title, abstract and keywords from 1800 journals having 47 million citations.

NGC (National Guideline Clearance House): indexes summaries of guidelines and links to full text versions.

Dissertation Abstracts: – a guide to US dissertations since 1861 and British dissertations for 50 universities since 1988.

Irrespective of the search engine/database, the information related to the content of the databases will usually be organised in similar ways. Bibliographic databases generally store publication information in the form of the title, author, book/journal title, year, journal volume, issue and page numbers. The full texts of articles are not always available on these databases. There has, however, been a growth in 'open access' publishing where research findings are made freely available, with databases such as the Directory of Open Access Journals providing information from over 1800 open access journals.

All databases have a help tab if you get into problems whilst using them. Many of the databases provide the facility to create your own 'workspace' where you can save previous searches and information for future use.

Finding the literature you want

In searching electronically, the words you have generated in relation to your PICO/ PICo question are used to form what is known as a **search filter**. A search filter is the information you put into the database to find the sources of evidence you want. These can be simple or complex – you will see in Chapter 9 that extensive filters are used in systematic reviews. Some databases have filters built into them, while in others you have to provide these yourself.

All databases use standard words to describe the content of articles, with the most well known being the medical subject headings commonly known as **MeSH terms**. Each database has its own thesaurus or index structure – CINAHL, for example, has 12,714 subject headings which it states reflects the language used by health professionals. If you type a word or phrase into a database usually it will offer you alternative terms: these are the subject headings. When searching you can decide whether to go with your own phrase or to use the subject headings provided. You can also search for exact phrases through the use of quotation marks – ' '/" ". If for instance you want to retrieve information in relation to essential skills clusters, this is placed in the search box as 'essential skills cluster', only publications containing the exact phrase are retrieved.

Activity

Type the text words you identified earlier into a database of your choice. What alternative terms are offered? Consider whether these more closely describe you area of interest.

An alternative method of identifying subject headings, known as **citation pearl growing**, is offered by Stott (1999). In this scenario you locate an article related to your area of interest that you already know (the pearl) and look at the subject headings on the retrieved record – these are usually found by 'clicking' on the full/complete reference link on the database. Those that appear relevant are used to locate similar articles, and the subject headings within them considered and added to the search strategy. If you don't have a 'pearl' to start with you can simply use your text words and then review the subject headings of the article records that are retrieved.

Databases give you the option of searching using keywords or authors' names. You may also be aware that a particular expert has written widely on a particular topic. If so, you may want to start by searching for literature written by that individual and looking at the subject headings used in relation to relevant articles by him/her.

Most databases also offer a 'related article' tab. This will allow you to access similar articles to any article of interest found. This can be useful in tracking down further relevant articles, however it must be used with care as it is very easy to get sidetracked into areas that are related to, but not specifically about your chosen topic.

In choosing a subject heading you may be offered two further options – to focus or explode the heading. If you choose to focus the heading a series of subheadings are given and you can restrict the search to certain areas. The articles that have the subheading(s) as their main focus are retrieved. See Box 5.4 for an example of the focus terms generated for the subject heading 'learning disabilities'.

Box 5.4   Focus terms associated with the search term 'learning disabilities' from MEDLINE database in 2012

Blood	
Cerebrospinal fluid	Metabolism
Chemically induced	Microbiology
Classification	Mortality
Complications	Nursing
Diagnosis	Parasitology
Diet therapy	Pathology
Drug therapy	Physiopathology
Economics	Prevention & control
Enzymology	Psychology
Epidemiology	Radiography
Ethnology	Radionuclide imaging
Etiology	Rehabilitation
Genetics	Therapy
History	Urine
Immunology	Virology

If you chose the 'explode' option it will provide a series of headings associated with the selected term which you can also include in your search. For instance the CINAHL thesaurus tree in relation to leg ulcer is:

Skin and connective tissue disease
  Skin disease
    Skin ulcer
      Fungating wound
      Leg ulcer
        Foot ulcer
        Venous ulcer
          Pressure ulcer
            Pyoderma gangrenosum

If you explode the search all items including the term 'leg ulcer' and those listed below it will be retrieved.

Boolean terms

These are the words *'and'*, *'or'* and *'not'* which are used to combine search terms. So for example if you are interested in literature related to Alzheimer's disease, you many consider using the terms Alzheimer's and dementia. A search of MEDLINE using the Boolean terms generated the following results:

- Dementia *and* Alzheimer's – 16,468 articles containing both words.
- Dementia *or* Alzheimer's – 117,166 articles containing either of the terms.
- Dementia *not* Alzheimer's – 57,188 articles containing dementia and not Alzheimer's.

Clearly if you want articles related to dementia and Alzheimer's then the use of 'and' is the best option. However if you are interested in dementia generally but not Alzheimer's specifically, then 'not' might be the most appropriate term to use.

Truncation

Truncation allows you to search for words that may appear in various forms, without having to include them all in the search. It entails the use of truncation marks (often $ or *) after a stem word. Rather than looking for fall, falls, falling you could simply put fall* or falls$. However, the down side is that this type of searching generates lots of results as any passing reference to the word is retrieved. For example when I searched CINAHL for dementia and fall* 558 records of publications were returned, but when I looked at the first 10 results two articles focusing on dementia had been retrieved that were irrelevant. One because of the author's name – Fallon – and another because the abstract included the term 'fall into line'.

Wildcards

Where words may have various spellings – such as paediatric and pediatric – a symbol (often ?) can be placed in the word at the point where the variation may occur. In this case you would use 'p?ediatric'. Words with that spelling will be then searched for and retrieved.

Limiting

Most databases allow you to limit your search in certain ways once your free text and/or subject headings have been accepted. You can limit your search in terms of publication dates – choosing a particular year or span of years. This can be useful if you are interested in the most recent information about a topic. Other limits include language – you can choose to include only English articles in the search; or full text – only those available to you as full text are retrieved; and/or patient group, which would include child, adult, etc. Databases allow you to limit your search to particular forms of evidence – research papers, reviews, meta-analysis, etc.

Searching for evidence

When searching for literature there are a few simple steps that will help you with the process:

1 Find out what databases are available to you through your education institution or health organisation.
2 Familiarise yourself with the databases and how they work – what subject heading, search filters, truncation and wildcard symbols, etc. are used in each.
3 Identify your search terms – be exact about what it is you want to find.
4 Put your search terms into the database you feel is most appropriate, using Boolean terms, truncation and/or wildcards as appropriate.
5 Focus, explode and/or limit your search as appropriate.
6 Examine the retrieved items for relevant literature. If a particularly relevant article is retrieved examine its subject headings to identify if you have missed any relevant areas from your own search.

Once you have practised a few times, then the process will become easier and you will find locating relevant literature an easier task.

Managing the evidence

Once you have gone through the search process you will have a list of documents that the database has identified as matching your search parameters. If there are a large number of results you may want to consider increasing the limiters you use – possibly in terms of publication dates, type of document, or full text only. The larger the list the longer it will take you to go through it.

The literature will usually be presented in the format of title of article, author(s), journal title, issue number, year of publication and language. A 'complete reference' tab is generally available – if clicked this will display all information about the article including abstract, if available, and the MeSH/subject headings under which the article was filed. If the abstract is available there will also be an 'abstract' tab which enables you to view the abstract only. Now you will need to go through the articles to identify if any/all are relevant to your area of interest. The easiest way to do this is scan the abstracts. From these you should be able to tell what is and is not appropriate. Most databases include facilities to save, print, email or export to bibliography software programmes such as EndNote. This is a useful tool as it helps you to keep track of what you want to read, create reference lists and find/order articles from library services at a later date. Where full text articles are available, you will often be able to download these to your computer as PDFs.

EBP Activity

Identify a problem related to your clinical area of practice and using the 'Forming a Question and Searching for Evidence' template in Appendix 3 to generate a question. Using the steps identified locate three papers relevant to your focus.

Summary

- Four resources are available to make decisions about integrating evidence into practice – systems, synopses, syntheses in the form of systematic reviews and original studies.
- Searching for evidence is a skill that takes time and practice to develop and librarians can be a key resource in finding the information you need.
- It is important to be aware of what resources are available to you when searching for evidence.
- All databases use standard words to describe the content of articles – known as subject headings – the most well known are the medical subject headings – MeSH terms. Free text and/or MeSH/subject headings can provide the means to locating relevant literature.
- Boolean terms, truncation and wildcards help you to streamline your search and ensure relevant literature is found.

Further reading

Czaplewski, L.M. (2012) 'Searching the literature: A researcher's perspective', *Journal of Infusion Nursing*, 35(1): 20–26. Gives an easy to understand account of how to search for literature.

Greenhalgh, T. (2006) *How to Read a Paper: The Basics of Evidence-Based Medicine* (3rd edn). Oxford: Blackwell. Provides an excellent chapter on searching for evidence.

Stillwell, S.B., Fineout-Overholt, E., Melnyk, B.M. and Williamson, K.M. (2010) 'Searching for evidence', *American Journal of Nursing*, 110(5): 41–47. For further exploration of approaches to locating evidence.

E-resources

CETL Reusable Learning Objects: this website provides reusable learning objects (RLOs) related to a range of topics. These are multimedia overviews of various topics. The study skills section contains an RLO related to conducting a literature search. www.rlo-cetl. ac.uk/index.php

Directory of Open Access Journals: provides information related to articles published in open access journals. www.doaj.org/

Greynet: provides open access to 7,000,000 references to grey literature. www.greynet.org

Evidence Update: reviews, critically appraises and rates articles from over 120 journals. Registration is free. http://group.bmj.com/products/evidence-centre/evidence-updates

Conclusion to Part 1

The aim of this section was to provide you with an underpinning knowledge of the various aspects of evidence-based practice and the skills associated with the first three aspects of the process as identified in Chapter 1. That is:

- the ability to identify what counts as appropriate evidence;
- forming a question to enable you to find evidence for consideration;
- developing a search strategy;
- finding the evidence.

This section ends with a crossword puzzle, with clues to answers relevant to Chapters 1, 2, 3, 4 and 5. The answers can be found on p. 177.

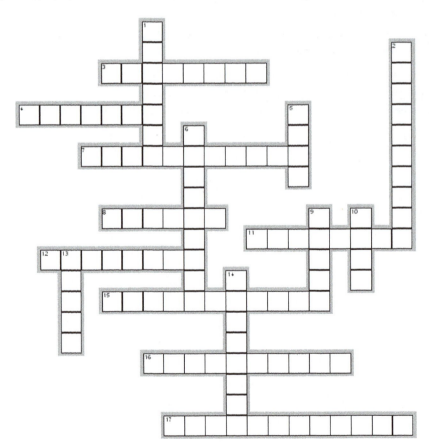

Across

3 information on which to base best practice? (8)

4 words used to combine search terms? (7)

7 items of evidence grouped together to provide a greater effect? (11)

8 theorist's surname – proposed a framework of nursing knowledge? (6)

11 set of logically connected ideas? (8)

12 central point for storing information in relation to specific topics? (8)

15 considering implications of decisions over time? (11)

16 belief that only what can be observed can be called fact? (10)

17 belief that humans actively construct their reality? (12)

Down

1 a body of knowledge organised in a systematic way? (7)

2 the belief that reality is ordered and can be studied objectively? (10)

5 terms used to describe medical subject headings? (4)

6 essential aspect of clinical decision making? (9)

9 knowledge used by practitioners drawn from experience? (5)

10 format for creating search questions? (4)

13 process for gathering information to promote effective care? (5)

14 last name of the 'father' of EBM? (8)

Part 2

Critiquing the Evidence

6

What is Critical Appraisal?

Learning Outcomes

By the end of the chapter you will be able to:

- define critical appraisal and its role in EBP;
- discuss the components of critical appraisal in relation to different forms of evidence;
- describe the skills of critical appraisal;
- locate appropriate critical appraisal tools.

Introduction

Critical appraisal is a key component of EBP and as such a core skill for those engaged in EBP. Much of what is written in relation to this area relates to critical appraisal of published research literature. However the types of evidence available are increasing, particularly in the form of clinical guidelines. It is essential that you critically appraise all evidence before integrating it into your practice. In this chapter therefore various issues related to critical appraisal and what this means in relation to journal articles and clinical guidelines are considered. Examples of tools that can help you with this process are identified and the skills you need to develop outlined.

So what is critical appraisal?

According to the Collins Dictionary (1998) critical means 'containing careful or analytical evaluation' and appraisal is 'an assessment or estimation of worth, value or quality of a thing'. Therefore critical appraisal can be said to be a careful evaluation of the worth, value or quality of evidence. It is not just about the identifying of weaknesses in a piece of evidence but also about noting the strengths – critical appraisal should be an objective consideration of the merits and limitations of the evidence.

When critically appraising something, Buckingham et al. (2008) suggest there are three central issues to be considered:

1　Validity – do you think the information is trustworthy?
2　Clinical importance – will this information make a difference to the quality/effectiveness of care?
3　Applicability – is it useable in your specific practice context?

The end result of critical appraisal should be a balanced consideration of a study's validity and significance for practice, this will help you make decisions as to how best to incorporate appropriate findings into your practice.

Critical appraisal of research literature

Parkes et al. (2001: 1) defined critical appraisal as 'the process of assessing and interpreting evidence by systematically considering its validity, results and relevance to an individual's work'. They suggest that a basic understanding of research methods is essential when undertaking critical appraisal. It is therefore important that you develop a basic knowledge of the research process and its various components.

One of the problems with published work is people assume that because something is in print it must be 'good' evidence, but this may not be so. Although most research papers are subject to some sort of peer review process – where other people have scrutinised the work and commented on its appropriateness for publication – not all published work is of a good standard. Even when research is of good quality, most studies will still have some methodological weaknesses, as Nieswiadomy (2008) identified; there is no such thing as a perfect research study, all have flaws or limitations of some sort. If research findings are to be used in practice it is vital you are aware of these limitations and consider their implications for introducing evidence into your clinical area.

Polit and Beck (2008) have noted that frequently there are 'grey areas' in relation to some aspects of research, with experts having different opinions as to what they believe to be appropriate when conducting a study. As research methodologies develop and studies progress, researchers have to weigh up the differing opinions and issues relating to their area of interest and then make decisions about how to proceed with the research. This then has an impact on the overall research outcomes. There are often compromises to be made in terms of what is considered ideal and what is practicable in the given situation. These compromises are often related to issues such as sample sizes, the methods used to collect and analyse data and/or the interpretation of findings. When critically appraising work you evaluate these decisions asking questions such as, 'Would another approach have been better?', 'Does the form of analysis have implications for the findings?' or 'Was the sample size sufficient to justify their conclusions?' and should then decide if these have implication for the study as a whole and its relevance for your practice.

Issues related to the **validity, reliability, trustworthiness** and **relevance** of research studies are of prime importance to critical appraisal (D'Auria, 2007) and all of these concepts will be considered in more depth in later chapters. Briefly, however, validity relates to whether or not the claims made in a study are accurate; so for instance if the paper suggests its findings are generalisable, there is a need to consider if the methodology used supports such a claim. Reliability is concerned with identifying if the results are dependable and replicable and involves asking the question, 'If the research was repeated would the same results be found?' The concept of trustworthiness relates to whether data can be considered dependable and credible. Finally, relevance is seen as a consideration as to whether the findings can be applied to the practice setting. Although these concepts are relevant to all forms of research, different criteria are often needed to make these judgements in relation to different research paradigms.

Quantitative research will tend to be judged in terms of reliability and validity whereas qualitative approaches generally focus more on **credibility, dependability, confirmability** and **transferability** (see Chapter 8 will deal with these concepts). However both sets of criteria are based on the idea of **rigour**, which involves a judgement as to whether the research is of a high quality and whether measures were in place to ensure that the research was conducted in an appropriate way, consistent with the underpinning principles associated with the research paradigm.

Published research papers do tend to have a specific form, being divided into particular sections. In critical appraisal each of these sections is examined and certain aspects of each section are considered. The format of papers may vary slightly from journal to journal or appear in a different order when certain research approaches are used. Generally the content remains the same, with all the aspects appearing in some form. There are, however, concerns about the quality of the reporting of research studies in journals. The EQUATOR (Enhancing the Quality and Transparency of Health Research) network has been set up to facilitate the development of reporting guidelines, which it is hoped will improve transparency of studies and the accuracy of reporting. These have been created mainly for the use of authors, journal editors and peer reviewers and most researchers now use these approaches in designing and writing up their research studies. These guidelines can also make critical appraisal much easier.

Activity

Identify a topic of interest related to your recent clinical experience. Find two research articles related to the topic – one using a qualitative and one using a quantitative approach. Compare the articles' sections, identifying the similarities and the differences. Visit the EQUATOR website at www.equator-network.org/home/ and identify if there are guidelines related to your chosen articles' methodology. If so, consider whether the articles meet the criteria identified.

A framework to critique research is offered by Polit and Hungler (1989) which identifies the broad areas that should be considered in critical appraisal and relevant to all forms of research (see Table 6.1). Parahoo (2006) suggests that the over-arching issues of sources of bias and omissions/exaggeration also need to be considered. Bias is a distortion of the results and/or conclusions and can be introduced in a number of ways – from the participants, the researcher(s), methods of data collection, the environment and the phenomena under study. These will be considered in more depth in relation to qualitative and quantitative approaches in the following chapters.

Table 6.1 Elements for critique

Dimension	Issues to be considered
Substantive/theoretical	• Is this an important area to study? • Does it have relevance to practice? • Does it take knowledge in this area forward? • Does the research approach fit with the question to be answered?
Methodological	• Are the research design, sampling method, data collection tool and forms of analysis rigorous and appropriate to the research question/hypothesis?
Practical	• Is the scope of the proposed research too broad? • Have practical issues related to the actually 'doing' of the research been given consideration?
Ethical	• Has the researcher identified the ethical issues associated with the research? • Has ethical approval been sought and given?
Interpretive	• Is the researcher's interpretation of the findings credible in light of the data? • Does the researcher's interpretation appear logical when compared with your own understanding of the area and other research on the topic?
Presentation/style	• Is there enough information? • Is it presented in a clear and concise way? • Are the themes and arguments developed in a logical and reasoned way?

Exaggeration tends to be in the form of writers over-emphasising the relevance of certain results. For example, if you asked people whether they preferred jam or marmalade on their toast and 46 per cent said jam, you could say almost half of the people preferred jam, or fewer than half preferred jam, each statement implies something different in relation to the same result. Omissions generally fall into two categories – intentional and unintentional. The former is serious if there is an intention to deceive the reader by deliberately leaving out information that may identify flaws in the work. The latter are the most common and often a result of researchers being so familiar with their work that they forget that others may not have the same level of understanding. This often results in aspects of the study not being clearly explained or described. Also, in writing for publication, researchers will commonly experience problems in terms of the article length. Journals allow authors a fixed number of words which may result in certain aspects being left out or minimal description being included. This is a particular problem in qualitative research where the data collected are generally in the form of words, all of which might not be included in the article.

Activity

Examine the two papers you chose for the preceding activity and identify any potential examples of exaggeration and/or omission in the papers. Consider the implications this might have in relation to the applicability of the studies to practice.

It is important to identify a study's methodology before you begin to critically appraise an article so that you can find an appropriate appraisal tool to help with the process. There are a large number of tools available both in books and on-line. For instance the NHS Public Health Resource Unit (2007) created a number of tools as part of its Critical Appraisal Skills Programme (CASP) aimed at promoting EBP. CASP tools are currently available for the critical appraisal of:

- systematic reviews;
- RCTs;
- qualitative research;
- economic evaluation;
- cohort studies;
- case control studies;
- diagnostic test studies.

Activity

Identify the methodological approach used in each of your chosen research studies. Find an appropriate appraisal tool for each of the studies.

Although qualitative and quantitative approaches are seen as different they do have some common areas for consideration which are discussed below. Appendix 4 provides a tool containing general criteria to consider when critiquing an article in this way.

Research design

The research design is the overall plan for the research and should be coherent and appropriate to the topic under consideration. One particular area for consideration is that of service user involvement. Just as there is increasing emphasis on the need to ensure the service user's voice is heard in the organisation and delivery of care, so too is user involvement becoming central to the research process, and this is not simply as participants but rather as part of the whole process. It is suggested that user involvement can generally occur at three levels (Grant and Ramcharan, 2006):

1   Consultation – users are consulted in relation to the appropriate issues to be considered and the design of the study.
2   Collaboration – service users are activity involved in the research process via recruiting participants, consent issues and collecting data.
3   User control – the research is conducted and controlled by service users.

Literature review

A review of literature relevant to a piece of the research is usually present in some form. It should be up-to-date, mainly from primary sources and relevant to the research question/hypothesis and proposed objective/aims. Parahoo (2006) suggests four criteria by which to judge a literature review:

1   Does it provide a rationale for the study? The review should identify why it is important the study is undertaken, the benefits and possible outcomes.
2   Does it put the current study into context? It should consider what is already known about the concepts under consideration and provide a balanced view of the various debates around the chosen focus.
3   Does it provide a review of research relevant to the topic? Research previously conducted should be considered and conclusions drawn, and implications for the proposed study identified.
4   Does it provide a conceptual/theoretical framework for the research? As you will see below not all research identifies a theoretical and conceptual framework, however a literature review should provide an overview of the different frameworks available.

Theoretical/conceptual framework

The purpose of research is to generate new knowledge, which involves the testing, adjusting and developing of theories. Therefore there is a need to identify what theory underpins or how it guides the research being critiqued. The terms theoretical framework and conceptual framework are often used interchangeably, although there are distinctions between them – the former usually refers to the use of one theory whereas the latter generally entails the combining of concepts from a range of theories. As Parahoo (2006) has pointed out, in practice this distinction is not always recognised by researchers. In fact this aspect is frequently missing from research reports or only mentioned in passing, particularly within quantitative research. It may, however, remain implicit within the literature review, the operational definitions or the discussion of the findings in relation to other literature.

Ethical issues

The Research Governance Framework for Health and Social Care states that 'the dignity, rights, safety and well-being of participants must be the primary consideration in any research study' (DH, 2005b: 7). All health service research undertaken in UK care organisations has required formal ethical approval since the Research Governance Framework became law in 2004. The DH (2005b: 7) requires research involving 'patients, service users, care professionals, volunteers, organs, tissue and data to be reviewed independently to ensure it meets ethical standards'. The regulations governing other countries may vary but the underlying principles are generally the same, reflecting the World Medical Association's (2004) Declaration of Helsinki concerning the ethical principles health professionals should consider (see www.wma.net/en/30publications/10policies/b3/index.html). Although not legally binding the declaration has been a major influence of the development of legislation relating to research ethics across the world.

Population

The population is the particular group of people that a researcher is interested in. It could be people with a learning disability who have challenging behaviour or children between the ages of 10 and 16 years who have appendicitis. It refers to the entire group; however data are not usually collected from the whole of a particular population.

Sampling

This term describes the segment of the identified population selected to take part in the study. People who form the sample within quantitative research are generally termed **subjects** or **sampling units**. Generally the word **participant** is used in relation to those who take part in qualitative research. This reflects the basic philosophy that individuals take an active role in the research process, rather than being passive subjects. Different ways of identifying the sample are used in qualitative and quantitative research and are discussed in more detail in Chapters 7 and 8.

Pilot study

Often before the full research study is carried out, a small 'pilot' study will be conducted to test out the design and forms of data collection. This allows for any adjustments to be made to the main study if there are problems with certain aspects. For example, the questions in a questionnaire may be changed if they are found to be unclear or ambiguous when tested on a small group first.

Data collection, analysis and results

These areas relate to what type of information is to be collected, how it will be gathered, processed, analysed and reported. This will be discussed in more depth in the following chapters.

Discussion

Polit and Beck (2008) have argued that the discussion should address the main findings of the study and what they mean, consider evidence to support the validity of the findings and examine what limitations may impact on this validity. There is also a need to consider the findings in light of what is already known and to then draw conclusions as to the usefulness of these to practice.

Applicability to practice

Finally, applicability relates to whether research findings can be applied to a setting. To judge applicability sufficient information must be present within the evidence to identify whether the population sampled in the study is comparable with the population that you identified in the clinical literature review question. Information related to age, cultural beliefs and values, ethnicity and lifestyle is essential if a judgement is to be made. As with any form of research whilst there may be evidence that a particular treatment is effective, there is still a need to consider it in light of specific patient preferences in an area of practice.

Critiquing clinical guidelines

Clinical guidelines are being generated everywhere and now seem readily available on almost any topic. Field and Lohr (1990: 38) defined guidelines as 'systematically developed statements to assist practitioners and patient decisions about appropriate health care'. Although guidelines have been around for a long time, recently they have become an important aspect of clinical governance and are seen as promoting clinical and cost effectiveness and providing a bridge between research and practice.

Whilst clinical guidelines are a useful aid to increasing the use of research in the delivery and management of care, they are not without problems. Bugers et al. (2002), for example, reviewed 15 clinical guidelines from 13 countries on type 2 diabetes. Although there was overall general agreement in terms of management of the disease, some differences in terms of treatment were identified. They found that the guidelines' recommendations shared little common evidence, with only 1 per cent of evidence appearing in six or more of the guidelines. This lack of common ground highlights the need to give careful consideration to guidelines before using them in practice.

Sanderlin and Abdul Rahhim (2007) have offered guidance for critiquing clinical practice guidelines, suggesting that whilst these are important tools in promoting EBP there are various issues to be considered before implementing them. These relate to:

- strength of evidence;
- objective approach to development of guidelines;
- homogeneity of studies – based on studies that have similar designs and complementary results;
- whether study subjects are significantly similar to the relevant patient group;
- whether the guidelines are based on evidence that has been appropriately appraised.

In an effort to address these issues, processes for guideline development are being generated to ensure that they are produced in a rigorous and appropriate manner.

Many organisations now request that in compiling clinical guidelines developers use the Grades of Recommendation, Assessment, Development and Evaluation (GRADE) process (see www.gradeworkinggroup.org/). This approach provides guidance on how to rate the quality of evidence and strength of recommendations. It is seen as providing a 'systematic and transparent framework' for developing guidelines (Guyatt et al., 2011: 380). Guidelines produced using the grade approach indicate whether recommendations are based on strong or weak evidence and therefore give an indication of the merits of the evidence used. It may be helpful when critically appraising guidelines to identify whether or not the GRADE approach has been used.

The Appraisal of Guidelines Research and Evaluation Collaboration, now the AGREE Research Trust (www.agreetrust.org/), provides a tool for appraising clinical guidelines. This international collaboration's aim is to improve the quality and effectiveness of guidelines by promoting a common approach to their development and assessment. The AGREE tool was updated and AGREE II launched in 2009, consisting of 23 criteria organised in six domains. The AGREE Research Trust propose that the instrument can be used to assess all forms of guidelines (local, national, international) with the exception of quality guidance related to healthcare organisation issues, and provides a user's manual to help people with the process of appraisal.

Activity

Identify a set of guidelines you recently used in practice. Consider these against the AGREE II criteria at www.agreetrust.org/. Consider whether or not the guidelines meet the AGREE II criteria.

Skills of critical appraisal

It is important to remember that the skills of critical appraisal are developed over time, and as with most things the more you practise the easier it will get. Critically appraising something takes time; it shouldn't be a rushed activity as it requires you to read things carefully, checking the information provided, and possibly consulting other people and sources of information.

The first thing to consider is whether the evidence is from a credible source. If it comes from a journal there are generally some checks already in place – most journals will identify whether or not they subject submissions to peer review. As identified in Chapter 5 there are already some sources of pre-appraised evidence available. Internet sources do not always have such checks in place, for example self-publishing sites such as Wikis may have little or no control over the information placed on the web page or its trustworthiness. You will need to decide whether you believe the site to be credible, checking an organisation's credentials or asking others what they know about certain sites. Box 6.1 give some examples of what to look for when making a judgement as to a website's credibility. This may save you unnecessary work if you later find that the source is not reputable.

Box 6.1   Judging the credibility/reliability of a website

Check:

- the URL:

  - if it contains a tilde (~) this means it's been created by an individual and therefore is less likely to be credible;

- the domain name, e.g.

  - .com = commercial; may be biased;
  - .co.uk = commercial; may be biased;
  - .ac.uk = university; likely to be reliable;
  - .edu = education; likely to be reliable;
  - .gov = government; likely to be reliable.

- the site's publication/update date – the more recent the more likely it is to be accurate;
- the purpose of the site – is it trying to sell you something, if so it may be biased;
- contact details – these should be present, you may want to check authenticity of the group by 'googling' them for further details;
- is the site affiliated to an identified group (university, government, healthcare agency); if so it is likely to be more credible;
- the stated objective of the site – this may give an indication of the site's purpose and relevance to your area of interest;
- the information on the website – is it verified by other sources?
- the quality of writing – a large number of spelling/grammatical errors probably mean it's less reliable.

Greenhalgh (2006) has suggested beginning the actual appraisal process by 'getting your bearings' and asking three broad questions:

1   What clinical question is being answered?
2   What type of study is it?
3   Is the design appropriate to the area of research?

By asking these questions you can very quickly decide whether or not to continue with the appraisal of a particular piece of evidence. If the evidence doesn't address a question you are interested in, there is no point in continuing. Identifying the type of study enables you to find an appropriate tool to help you critique the work. The appropriateness of the approach is essential in answering your own clinical question. If you are interested in the effectiveness of an intervention but the approach used is one more suitable to considering the feasibility of using a particular intervention then, once again, there is no point in appraising the study. If the study meets all three of these criteria, then the next step it to undertake a full appraisal.

A similar approach known as 'Rapid Critical Appraisal' is put forward by Fineout-Overholt et al. (2010a). Here it is suggested you review studies to identify:

1   Type of study and place within the hierarchy of evidence.
2   How well it was conducted.
3   Applicability to practice.

In this approach a particular level of evidence is being looked, that is RCTs. Therefore the placing of the evidence within the hierarchy is essential. In steps 2 and 3 Fineout-Overholt et al. (2010b) advocated a consideration of the results and their validity and their relevance to the appraiser's own area of practice. Only if a paper meets the criteria related to appropriate level of evidence, valid results and apparent applicability to practice is it taken forward for full critical appraisal.

As was discussed in Chapter 5 there are sources of evidence that have already been appraised (DiCenso et al., 2009). It may also be useful to examine your search results to identify if any pre-appraised evidence has been found. Indeed if this is present and is at level 1, 2, 3 or 4 of DiCenso's hierarchy it may not be necessary to review the remaining literature.

To critically appraise evidence you need to take a step-by-step approach as outlined below, but as your confidence and skills grow you will develop your own system.

1   Identify a suitable checklist to use to critically appraise the evidence.
2   Find somewhere quiet, where you are unlikely to be interrupted.
3   Read through the paper once, so you have a grasp of the content.
4   Read through it again in more depth, evaluating each part of the paper.
5   Make notes or highlight important bits of the paper as you go along.
6   Have a research book to hand so you can check out information or fill in any gaps in your knowledge as you read.
7   Complete the appraisal and discuss your findings with others.

There are resources available to help develop skills in this area such as Critical Appraisal Topics (CATs). These are summaries of evidence relating to a clinical question generated in response to a specific clinical problem (Foster et al., 2001). Originally a paper-based exercise generated by McMaster University in Canada to encourage medical students to develop critical appraisal skills, CATs created by various individuals are available online as a possible resource and learning tool for other health professionals. An electronic tool known as a CAT-maker created by the NHS Research and Development Centre for Evidence-Based Medicine at Oxford is also freely available to help with the generation of your own CAT. Although this has been developed for the medical profession, the process can also be of use to others in the healthcare setting as it can provide a summary of the evidence and ends with a judgement as to its appropriateness to address the question asked.

Activity

Visit the Centre for Evidence-Based Medicine CAT-maker website at www.cebm.net/index. aspx?o=1216. Download the tool and consider whether this would be a useful tool in conducting your own critical appraisals.

CATs are a useful learning tool as they:

• provide an example of critical appraisal in relation to a live issue using accessible evidence sources;
• provide a concise step-by-step method for recording the process of critical appraisal which can then be shared with others;
• help in the development of critical appraisal skills;
• enable a structured and informed approach to clinical decision making.

However CATs are not without their disadvantages. They have a limited life span unless they are regularly updated and may contain errors due to a lack of individual knowledge or particular forms of interpretation.

It is useful to have an overview of the details of the literature you appraise, particularly if there are a number of studies you feel may be appropriate to your area of interest. The easiest way to do this is to generate a summary table of the various studies' details (see Appendix 5 for an example). This will be useful when you are later making decisions about integrating evidence into your practice.

In developing the skills associated with critical appraisal it is important to remember that to become proficient takes time and you are not expected to know everything or get it completely right the first time. It is important to know how to find the information you need to conduct the appraisal and to discuss your findings with others and ask for their opinions.

EBP Activity

Chose one of the papers you identified earlier. Using the appropriate critical appraisal tool undertake a critical appraisal of the paper identifying the aspects/questions you are able to fully critique and those where you need to develop further skills and knowledge. Develop an action plan outlining how you will develop the knowledge and skills you require to complete the task appropriately.

Summary

- Critical appraisal is associated with published research literature, but there is a need to appraise all forms of evidence.
- Critical appraisal should be an objective consideration of the merits and limitations of the evidence.
- Not all published work is of an appropriate standard or applicable to the practice setting, therefore critical appraisal is a key aspect of EBP.
- Skills of critical appraisal take time to develop and practice is essential.

Further reading

Fineout-Overholt, E., Melnyk, B.M., Stillwell, S.B. and Williamson, K.M. (2010) 'Critical appraisal of evidence: part 1', *American Journal of Nursing*, 110(7): 47–52.

Fineout-Overholt, E., Melnyk, B.M., Stillwell, S.B. and Williamson, K.M. (2010) 'Critical appraisal of evidence: part 2', *American Journal of Nursing*, 110(9): 41–48. Both these articles provide an overview of an approach to critical appraisal of evidence.

Parahoo, K. (2006) *Nursing Research: Principles, Process and Issues* (2nd edn). Basingstoke: Palgrave Macmillan. Provides an excellent introduction to the research process.

E-resources

Critical Appraisal Skills Programme: provides a range of resources to help with developing the skills associated with EBP. Also provides a range of critical appraisal tools. www.phru.nhs.uk/Pages/PHD/CASP.htm

National Institute for Clinical Excellence: provides national guidance on preventing and treating illness and promoting health. www.nice.org.uk

Netting the Evidence Google Search Engine: searches 107 sites associated with EBP. http://tinyurl.com/2poh3a

7

Critical Appraisal and Quantitative Research

Learning Outcomes

By the end of the chapter you will be able to:

- provide an overview of quantitative research approaches;
- identify the key areas for consideration when critically appraising quantitative literature;
- debate issues of reliability and validity.

Introduction

Quantitative research is primarily concerned with examining how different things known as variables interact and impact on each other. Florence Nightingale is said to have employed quantitative research methods by collecting statistical data during the Crimean War and saw statistics as a vital tool for ensuring healthcare was based on sound evidence. Mantzoukas (2008) found that 51 per cent of research studies published in the top 10 generic nursing journal (such as the *Journal of Advanced Nursing, Journal of Clinical Nursing*) were quantitative in nature.

As quantitative research involves 'numbers' and the use of statistics this often produces a 'panic' response in some people who feel they will not be able to understand the analysis. However, as Greenhalgh (2006) identifies, all you really need to know is what is the best test to apply in given circumstances, what is does and what might affect its validity/appropriateness. It is not necessary to understand the actual calculations involved.

In this chapter I intend to look at the methods used in quantitative research and discuss the issues you should consider when critically appraising. However, it is not my intention to provide a full overview of quantitative research, for a more in-depth exploration you will need to consider some of the recommended reading at the end of the chapter.

So what is quantitative research?

As identified in Chapter 2 quantitative research has its roots in positivism and in using a deductive approach, starting with a theoretical framework or conceptual model which predicts how things (**variables**) behave in the world. Specific predictions (**hypotheses**) are then deduced from the theory and tested (Polit and Beck, 2008). The aim of quantitative research is therefore to explore the relationships between variables and to test hypotheses. It is seen as using objective, rigorous and systematic approaches. A researcher will identify the variables of interest, clearly define what these are and then collect data usually in a numerical form.

A variable, simply put, is something that varies from one person/situation to another. So weight, temperature, pain, personality traits are all variables. Quantitative research seeks to understand why these variations occur. For example, in mental health, depression is a variable as not everyone experiences depression. It is possible to study what factors are linked with the onset of depression. If a variable is extremely varied within a particular group it is said to be heterogeneous and where there is limited variability it is described as being homogeneous. Table 7.1 outlines some different types of variables.

Table 7.1 Types of variables

Type	Description
Dependent	• The focus of the research • The characteristic or behaviour that the researcher is attempting to understand, describe or affect
Independent	• The factor/characteristic that is considered to have an influence on the dependent variable
Confounding	• A significant association between two variables occurs because of being associated with a third variable

Usually the relationship between independent variable and dependent variables will be considered. In mental health, for example, you could consider whether age (independent variable) has any implications for the onset of depression (dependent variable). Whether a variable is identified as dependent or independent depends on the focus of the study. In the above example depression is the dependent variable, however you could consider whether depression (independent variable) is associated with suicide (dependent variable).

Polit and Beck (2008) suggest quantitative research generally considers specific questions about the relationships, such as:

• The relationship between variables – e.g. is body weight related to the onset of type 2 diabetes?
• The direction of a relationship between variables – e.g. is someone who is overweight more or less likely to develop type 2 diabetes?

- The strength of the relationship between variables – e.g. how likely is it that someone who is overweight will develop type 2 diabetes?
- The cause and effect relationship between the variables – e.g. does being overweight cause the development of type 2 diabetes?

Usually a hypothesis is generated providing a simple statement of the variables to be considered and the relationship between them. For example, I could hypothesise that providing play activities (independent variable) for children prior to surgery will reduce their anxiety (dependent variable).

Activity

Consider an issue which is causing concern in your area of practice. Identify the variables that might be considered in a study and generate a hypothesis as to the relationship between them.

Usually a large number of people are used in quantitative research, therefore statistical tests are used to help make sense of the data and enable these to be presented in an understandable form. Statistics also help in making judgements regarding the value of research findings for the research population as a whole (i.e. is it generalisable?). Analysis is an attempt to measure the concepts and variables under consideration as accurately and objectively as possible. Objectivity is seen as a central tenet of quantitative research, with the researcher viewed as 'standing outside' the research process. The intention here is to ensure that neither the researcher nor the subjects introduce any form of bias into the research process. Bias is where the results of a study are distorted for some reason (this will be considered in more detail later in the chapter). To reduce bias a process known as blinding is often used. Here information relating to the research process is concealed from those on whom the research is conducted and/or those involved in delivering the intervention being studies. For example, if the effectiveness of a particular drug is being tested an experimental group of subjects receive the drug and a control groups receive a placebo. The subjects and/or those administering the drug may not be made aware of who is receiving the drug and who is receiving the placebo. If information is withheld from only one of the groups involved – the subjects or those administering the drug – it is called a single-blind study. If information is withheld from both groups it would be known as a double-blind study.

Types of quantitative research

Generally two types of research design are present within quantitative research: experimental and non-experimental.

Experimental approaches, with the most common in the healthcare setting being RCTs, actively introduce a treatment or intervention in an attempt to study causal relationships. The aim is to identify whether a particular intervention has an impact on the dependent variable. To be a true experimental design the following three conditions must be met:

1   An intervention is controlled by a researcher so some subjects receive the intervention and others don't – this is known as manipulation of the variable.
2   At least two groups of subjects are involved – a control group and an experimental group.
3   Random selection and allocation of subjects to research groups will occur.

If these three conditions are not all met, the research is described as quasi-experimental, with the most common unmet condition being the random assignment of subjects. Quasi-experimental approaches are used to test the effectiveness of interventions but are seen as less rigorous and often there is less confidence in the ability to generalise the findings.

Concerns have been raised in relation to the quality of the reporting of this type of research. It is suggested that frequently the information given is not sufficient to allow proper critical appraisal. To address these concerns guidelines as to what should be included in reports of RCTs have been generated, these are known as the CONSORT (Consolidated Standards of Reporting Trials) statement (CONSORT, 2012). Various 'extensions' to the CONSORT statement have been developed to give guidance on specific designs, data and interventions. Statements related to other forms of quantitative research are also being developed. These may be of help in identifying what should be included in quantitative research studies.

Activity

Visit the CONSORT website at www.consort-statement.org and identify the aspects that are considered to be central to the designing and writing up of randomised control trials (RCTs).

Non-experimental qualitative research is used to describe and/or identify associations between variables and would generally be used to address Polit and Beck's (2008) first three questions (see above) about relationships between variables. However there is no attempt to manipulate variables or to identify cause and effect relationships. Instead the intention is to observe what is happening without intervening. Often these designs are classified in terms of when the data collection occurs.

Cross-sectional studies will compare different groups within a population of interest, collecting data at a single point in time. For example if you wanted to measure whether the length of time someone was in residential care impacts on their level of satisfaction, you might collect data at the same point from individuals who had been in residence for three months, six months, nine months and twelve months and compare the findings.

Longitudinal studies will collect data at various points over an extended period of time from an identified individual/group of people. For example, if you were interested in the impact of socioeconomic factors on the health outcomes of children from birth to the age of six you would collect data from the same group of children from birth to the age of six years at defined intervals (perhaps at six-month intervals).

Retrospective studies collect data after an event. For example, patients' notes may be examined for information in relation to a specific treatment and recovery. Alternatively **prospective studies** collect data in relation to a specific independent variable and the dependent variable is measured at a later date. In this approach it would be possible, for example, to consider if coping behaviours in relation to stress have an impact on incidence of myocardial infarctions by measuring stress coping behaviours in a population and then identifying the number of people who had a myocardial infarction in 10 years' time.

The most common types of research design are in the form of **descriptive** and **correlation studies**. Descriptive studies generally observe, describe and document areas of interest as they occur naturally. Correlation studies are employed in the examination of relationships between variables, without manipulation of the independent variable. Table 7.2 provides a list of the different types of research you are likely to come across. Again, as identified in relation to RCTs, reporting guidelines have been created with regard to a number of these approaches and can be found at the EQUATOR network website (www.equator-network.org/home/).

Table 7.2 Types of quantitative research designs

Experimental	Non-experimental
Pre-test-post-test control group design	Surveys
Post-test-only control group design	Correlation
Solomon four-group design	Comparative
Non-equivalent control group design	Methodological
Times series design	Secondary analysis studies

Critical appraisal

As identified in Chapter 6, there are a number of tools available to help you critically appraise quantitative research. Appendix 6 gives a generic approach to particular areas to be addressed in this form of critique – those specific to quantitative research are highlighted, and an overview is given below. For discussion of the other general items see Chapter 6. Remember, when doing a critical appraisal it is helpful to have good research book to hand so you can check or clarify information as you go along.

Activity

Find a quantitative research study relevant to your area of practice and an appropriate critical appraisal tool.

Hypothesis/research question and research objectives/aims

Not all quantitative research has a hypothesis, particularly descriptive approaches. However, if this is not present there should be a clearly stated research question. If a hypothesis is required this should be a simple statement identifying the relationship between at least two clearly stated variables and should be testable. You will come across different types of hypotheses, including:

- Directional – this precisely indicates the nature and direction of the relationship between variables – *positive* (e.g. increased physical activity improves mental functioning); *inverse/ negative* (e.g. people with learning disabilities display less challenging behaviour when involved in diversional activities); *difference* (e.g. people with depression are more likely to commit suicide than those who are not depressed).
- Non-directional – this only identifies that a relationship exists (e.g. children differ from adults in the levels of anxiety they experience on admission to hospital).
- Null hypothesis – where no relationship is identified (e.g. there is no relationship between the use of cognitive behavioural therapy and an improvement of mood in people who are depressed).

The aims/objectives of the research should also be clearly identified and reflect the research question and/or hypothesis.

Operational definitions

It is expected that concepts used within the research will be defined. For example if a study related to whether wound dressing X is more effective than wound dressing Y in the treatment of leg ulcers, there is a need to clearly define what is meant by wound dressings X and Y, leg ulcer, the procedures to be used when applying the dressing and the effects to be measured. Whilst words such as 'leg ulcer' are in common usage, within the research context there is a need to identify precisely what type of leg ulcers are to be considered. Without this type of information the rigour and the generalisability of the findings can be called into question and the ability to identify if the research is relevant to your own area of practice is reduced.

Activity

Read the article chosen in the previous activity. Identify the operational definitions and appraise whether these are sufficiently described to allow you to identify applicability to your own area of practice.

Data collection methods

The measurement tools selected to collect data should be appropriate to the research question/hypothesis and the operational definitions and should also collect the type and level of data required. Data collection methods in quantitative research can take many forms – questionnaires, observational schedules, self-reporting schedules or biophysiological measures. All of these approaches involve the measurement of variables through the assignment of numbers to the variable according to identified rules. For example there are identified rules for measuring weight which allow you to observe what someone weighs and what is the accepted weight range in relation to height and age. However not all variables have measures already in place and these have to be created to allow measurement to be taken.

In considering measurement in quantitative research there is a need to understand:

1   What is being measured?
2   How it is being measured?
3   Why it is being measured in this way?
4   What the rules are in relation to that measurement?
    (Parahoo, 2006)

Without this information it is not possible to judge whether the data being collected can be trusted and appropriately represent the focus of the study.

There are two main criteria for assessing the research tools – reliability and validity – both are discussed in more detail below. However, briefly, reliability of measurement tools relates to the accuracy with which a tool is said to measure the variable, whether it is able to reproduce findings consistently and be free from error. Validity relates to whether the tool measures what it is said to measure. Frequently researchers use tools that have already been tested for reliability and validity. If a new tool is being used then there should be evidence that it has been pre-tested for its reliability/validity.

Data collection protocols are usually produced by quantitative researchers identifying procedures for collecting data. Clear instructions as to what conditions should be met and any specific instruction in relation to sequencing of collecting and recording of information are expected to be present.

Sampling

Studies almost always involve samples rather than the whole population of interest. If findings are to be generalised to the population of interest, then the sample must be seen as representative of the whole of that population. The sample size required for a particular study is often determined through the use of power calculations. Statistical power is the ability of a study to detect statistically significant results. The power of a test is affected by the sample size and power calculations will identify the sample size needed to detect significant differences where they exist. A well-designed study will identify the use of power calculations in calculating sample sizes.

Quantitative research generally uses what is known as probability sampling. In this type of sample every unit within the population of interest has an equal chance of being selected. To ensure representativeness random selection procedures are used. Appropriate randomisation is of central importance to an RCT as it is seen as ensuring that neither the researchers nor the subjects will be able to influence the outcomes of the study. Four approaches to probability sampling are available – simple, stratified, systematic and cluster (see Table 7.3).

Table 7.3 Types of randomised sampling

Type	Description
Simple random	• A sampling frame is generated listing all the elements of the population • A number is allocated to each one of the elements • A table of random grouped numbers (computer generated) is used to select sample units for specified sample size
Stratified random	• Ensures subgroups (e.g. age, ethnicity) within a population are present in sample in same proportions • **Proportional stratified sampling** = sample proportions are same as population • **Disproportional sampling** = a large sample of a particular subgroup is needed to consider the relationship between variables in that group • Weighting = adjustments made to statistical analysis to provide actual population values • Simple random sampling used to select the subjects from each subgroup
Cluster random (multi-stage) sampling	• Used in large-scale studies with a widespread geographical population • Clusters of target population randomly selected • Units within each cluster again randomly selected to be part of the sample • Simple random sampling would be used at each stage
Systematic random sampling	• Sample units are selected at predetermined intervals, e.g. every 5th or 7th or 20th unit on sampling frame • Interval used decided by dividing the available target population by the sample size required, e.g. 100 unit for a sample of 20 = every 5th unit selected (100 ÷ 20 = 5) • Sample frame itself is randomised before using this form of sampling

It is important that clear and precise accounts of the inclusion and exclusion criteria are documented within the study in order that the exact characteristics of the population used for the collection of data are known. Without this information, the generalisability of findings to other client groups will be called into question and therefore reduces your ability to make decisions as to the applicability of the research to your own area of practice.

Data analysis

Statistical analysis allows quantitative researchers to make sense of the mass of numbers generated in the collection of data. There are four levels of data within quantitative research – nominal, ordinal, interval and ratio (see Box 7.1). The level of data indicates the statistical test to be used. It is beyond the scope of this chapter to give a full account of all forms of data test and analysis and I strongly recommend that you identify a book that you can use to help you understand this aspect of the research process.

Box 7.1 Levels of data	
Scale	**Description**
Nominal	• Simply categorises groups (e.g. male or female) and assigns a code number to the identifying traits. Male = 1, Female = 2. • Allows the identification of the frequency of a trait within a category – for example identifying that 60 per cent of a sample were female.
Ordinal	• Codes information according to an order in relation to specified criteria. • Likert scales produce ordinal data (e.g. strongly agree, agree, disagree, strongly disagree).
Interval	• Rank ordering of characteristics, the distance between any two numbers on the scale is known (e.g. temperature scale).
Ratio	• Ordering of a trait, the intervals between each rank and the absolute magnitude of the trait (e.g. height or weight).

Zellner et al. (2007) having reviewed over 400 research articles in various nursing journals found that 80 per cent of these used the same 10 statistical approaches (see Box 7.2 for a description of these 10 approaches). In an evaluation of the statistical analysis presented in qualitative research from the top five nursing journals, Cohn et al. (2009) found 63 per cent of papers were descriptive or correlation surveys. It may be useful to familiarise yourself with these forms of statistical analysis as they are the ones you are most likely to come across.

Box 7.2   Description of statistical tests most commonly used in nursing research

Descriptive statistics

- Mean – the average sum of a set of values. If the ages of six people were identified as 26, 29, 30, 38, 40 and 41, the mean age would be 34 (26 +29 + 30 + 38 + 40 + 41 = 204 ÷ 6 = 34).

- Frequency distribution – the arrangement of data in ascending order (lowest to highest value), identifying the number of times a particular value or score occurs. If the stress levels of 50 people prior to surgery were measured and given a numerical score (ranging from 1 to 10) it might result in the following frequency distribution.

  Frequency 2 3 5 8 11 7 6 4 3 1 (n 50)

  Score   1 2 3 4 5 6 7 8 9 10

- Standard deviation – the average deviation of the values from the mean.

- Range – the distance between highest and lowest values and gives a picture of the dispersion of data (the range between 15 per cent and 85 per cent = 70).

- Percentages, percentiles and quartiles – the frequency at which something occurs is reported in percentages, e.g. 60 per cent of people prefer butter to margarine; a percentile is the point below which a specific percentage of values lies (a score at a 60th percentile means 60 per cent of scores are below that); quartiles divide distribution scores into four equal parts.

Inferential statistics

- t-test – examines the difference between the means of two sets of values.

- Analysis of variant (ANOVA) – examines the difference between several means.

- Correlation – identifies an association between variables where a variation in one is related to a variation in another.

- Cronbach's alpha – a reliability index used to measure internal consistency of a multi-itemed measurement tool such as an anxiety scale or an assessment tool.

- Chi-squared – compares data collected in the form of frequencies or percentages.

Briefly, statistics are identified as being either descriptive or inferential (Box 7.3 identifies the different types of descriptive and inferential statistics). Descriptive statistics, as the term suggests, 'describe' and summarise the data, often in the form of averages and percentages. Within the EBP movement one of the most useful forms of descriptive statistics in decision making are effect/risk measures. These measures are used to calculate the 'clinical meaningfulness' of findings and are frequently seen in systematic reviews. However, these are also being increasingly included in research reports and it may be useful for you to explore these in more depth (for a brief overview see Chapter 9).

Box 7.3 Types of descriptive and inferential analysis

Descriptive	Inferential	
	Parametric	*Non-parametric*
Frequency	Pearson	Chi-squared
Central tendency (mean, mode, median)		
Variability (range and standard deviation)	*t*-test	Mann-Whitney
Risk (absolute risk, absolute risk reduction, relative risk, relative risk ratio, odds ratio, numbers needed to treat)	ANOVA	Spearman's rho

Inferential statistics allow researchers to make 'inferences' (draw conclusions) about their findings and are usually divided into two types, parametric and non-parametric. The type of test used usually depends on:

- the sampling method;
- the level of data required (e.g. nominal);
- the distribution of variables to be measured.

Parametric tests are usually adopted where the sample is randomised, where the level of data is interval or ratio, and where there is a normal distribution of variables. These types of test are generally seen to be more powerful that non-parametric tests. Non-parametric tests do not consider a particular form of distribution to be present, and can be used with nominal and also ordinal data and on small samples.

Statistical tests that identify significance – whether an observed result is the product of chance or represents a finding of significance – are based on probability theory. This is commonly referred to as a p value, the smaller the p value the less likely the possibility that the result has occurred by chance. It is usually expressed as $p < 0.05$ (the symbol < identifies it is as less than; > would signify more than). Significance levels of 0.05, 0.01 and 0.001 are the most commonly cited p values in relation to significance of findings. A value of 0.05 identifies that the results are significant at a 5 per cent level, meaning that there is a less than five chances in a hundred (or 1 in 20) likelihood that the result has occurred by chance. The p value of 0.05 is generally accepted as the level at which it is possible to claim a positive result. There are two commonly used tests used to consider significance – chi-squared and t-test:

- the chi-squared test identifies significance between groups;
- the t-test identifies differences between groups.

Where statistical significance is identified usually *confidence intervals* are calculated to work out how precise the results are. The wider the interval, the less likely the same results would be found if the research was to be repeated a number of times. If you found that wound dressing X improved wound healing in 65 per cent of the sample, there is a need to know how precise that estimate is if it is to be applied to the wider population. The sample result is unlikely to be exactly the same as the population response to the treatment. It is possible to calculate an interval (with an upper and lower limit) in relation to the sample result that suggests the range within which the target population response to treatment will fall. If the confidence interval had a lower limit of 25 per cent and a higher limit of 100 per cent, the confidence interval is very wide and therefore the value of 65 per cent is very imprecise. If, however, the confidence interval is between 60 and 70 per cent, the estimate of 65 per cent is more precise and more meaningful. By convention researchers usually report confidence intervals of 95 per cent (expressed as 95 per cent CI), which are the range of values (the interval) within which there is 95 per cent confidence that the real value applies to the total population of patients.

Findings

It is usually the norm that descriptive statistics are presented first, to give the readers an overview of the variables. Findings are then generally ordered in terms of importance or in relation to the sequencing of the research question/hypotheses. Tables are used where a number of statistical tests are reported. Tables should be presented in a clear and easily understandable manner, with clear links to the written narrative. All data should be accounted for.

Reliability, validity and applicability

Reliability relates to the accuracy and consistency of findings, that whether the same results would be reached if the same variables were repeatedly measured in the same way (Bowling, 2009). For example, you may be fairly sure that a thermometer will accurately measure your temperature and that it would give the same results if you repeated the measurement at five-minute intervals. If two results varied by five degrees, you would question the reliability of the thermometer. In critically appraising research you are considering whether the research design, methodology and measurement tools provide accurate findings and whether, if you repeated the research in your own area, you could be sure that the same result would be found.

Validity is described by Polit and Beck (2008) as a property of inference. Researchers can only infer that a perceived effect is a result of their hypothesised case if the research is valid, namely that there is confidence that what was intended to be measured has been measured. Four types of validity are proposed by Polit and Beck:

1 Statistical conclusion validity – where tests are deemed to be appropriate/fair and any identified statistical relationship between the variables is based on sound evidence.
2 Internal validity – where a relationship is proven that this is the result of the independent variable, not some other circumstance, such as chance, confounding variables, introduction of bias, etc. (see Table 7.4).
3 Construct validity – relates to the degree a tool measures the thing it is designed to measure. For instance, you may be fairly sure that thermometer is a valid tool to measure temperature (unless it's broken in some way) but you might be less sure of a tool designed to measure pain.
4 External validity – concerns the generalisability of findings to other people and/or settings.

Table 7.4 Sources of bias

Type	Description
Selection bias	Inadequate randomisation
Performance bias	Differences in the way intervention is received/delivered
Attrition bias	More subjects are lost from one research group than another (control or experimental)
Detection bias	Differences which occur when assessing outcomes or RCTs
Participant bias	A lack of full disclosure or giving what is considered to be appropriate responses
Conceptual bias	Faulty conceptualisation of problem, interpretation of findings or drawing of conclusions
Design bias	Faults in any aspect of the research design
Recall bias	Difficulties relating to recalling of past events, memory degeneration over time

Table 7.5 Factors which may impact on validity

Type of validity	Threats to validity
Statistical conclusion	• Sample size is small • Tools lacking the precision to accurately measure the variables • Variations in the implementation of an intervention • Treatment adherence
Construct validity	• Hawthorne or placebo effect – people's behaviour as a response to being observed or to treatment because they believe it will have a positive effect • Researcher's response to subjects encourages certain responses • Novelty effect – perception of new treatments may result in positive or negative responses from subjects • Compensation – control group subjects are 'compensated' in some way by health staff or family for not receiving research intervention • Contamination – control and experimental group receive similar services generally or experimental group member moves to control group by dropping out of the trial

Table 7.5 gives an overview of some of the issues that threaten validity in relation to the above items.

Validity can also be compromised by confounding variables. As discussed earlier, confounding variables are where a proposed relationship between two variables may actually be due to a third variable. In critically appraising studies you must consider whether the researcher has considered potential confounding variables in the research design and analysis of the findings.

EBP Activity

Chose and locate a quantitative article of interest and critically appraise it using the questions in Appendix 6. Identify aspects where you need to develop further skills and knowledge. Then develop an action plan outlining how you will develop the knowledge and skills you require to complete the task appropriately.

Summary

• The aim of quantitative research is to explore relationships between variables and test hypotheses. The researcher identifies the variables of interest, clearly defines what these are and then collects data usually in a numerical form.
• The relationship between independent variables and dependent variables are considered. Statistics help in making judgements and generalisations

> of the value of the research findings for the research population as a whole.
> - Two types of research design are present within quantitative research: experimental and non-experimental.
> - Quantitative research generally uses what is known as probability sampling.
> - There are four levels of data within qualitative research – nominal, ordinal, interval and ratio. The level of data indicates the statistical test to be used.

Further reading

Bowling, A. (2009) *Research Methods in Health* (3rd edn). New York: Open University Press. Gives a good introduction to research and its use in the healthcare setting.

Greenhalgh, T. (2006) *How to Read a Paper: The Basics of Evidence-Based Medicine* (3rd edn). Oxford: Blackwell. Provides a number of critical appraisal tools and an easy to read chapter on 'Statistics for the non-statistician'.

Polit, D.F. and Beck, C.T. (2008) *Nursing Research: Generating and Assessing Evidence for Nursing Practice* (8th edn). Philadelphia: Lippincott Williams and Wilkins. Gives a good introduction to the various aspects of quantitative research and its approaches.

E-resources

CETL Reusable Learning Objects: this website provides reusable learning objects (RLOs) related to a range of topics. These are multimedia overviews of various topics. The 'EBP' and 'Statistics' sections contain RLOs related to the content of this chapter. www.rlo-cetl. ac.uk/index.php

CONSORT website: provides explanations and examples of what is expected to be included in some forms of quantitative research. www.consort-statement.org

Netting the Evidence Google Search Engine: searches 107 sites associated with EBP. http:// tinyurl.com/2poh3a

8

Critical Appraisal and Qualitative Research

Learning Outcomes

By the end of the chapter you will be able to:

- discuss qualitative research and its basic traits;
- list qualitative forms of data collection;
- identify the key areas for consideration when critically appraising qualitative literature;
- identify criteria used for evaluating the rigour of such studies.

Introduction

Qualitative research has been particularly used in the social sciences – sociology, psychology and anthropology – and many of the healthcare professions – nursing, pharmacy and social work. In the past there has been great debate, and at times furious disagreement, about the validity of qualitative approaches, which have often been criticised as being subjective, biased and lacking in generalisability. In earlier times qualitative and quantitative research approaches were seen as diametrically opposed. More recently, however, most people would agree that it is important to choose an approach that will provide the most appropriate answer to the question posed. Many research studies now adopt mixed methods, where qualitative and quantitative approaches are used side by side to address the issues under consideration. Mantzoukas (2008) identified that of the nursing research published in the top 10 generic nursing journals (such as the *International Journal of Nursing*) 37 per cent used qualitative methodologies and 2 per cent were mixed methods.

This chapter considers the methods and approaches used in qualitative research and discusses the issues you should consider when critically appraising literature of this type. However, as with the previous chapter, it is not my intention to provide a full overview of research process, and for a more in-depth explanation you need to consider some of the recommended reading at the end of the chapter.

So what is qualitative research?

As discussed in Chapter 2 qualitative research represents a different research paradigm to quantitative research. It has different philosophical underpinnings which give rise to different ways of thinking about the nature of knowledge and how this can be generated. Qualitative research focuses on words, how people describe their experiences, perspectives, understanding and beliefs/values. The words collected may be in spoken or written form. Qualitative research is an attempt to provide what is termed as a **thick** or **rich description** of the phenomenon from an **emic** (individual's) perspective rather than an **etic** (outsider's, or researcher's, perspective): namely, to give a full and thorough account of the research context, the meanings people attach to their experiences, their interpretation of issues and also what motivates them to behave/respond in particular ways. Qualitative research is seen as being holistic, giving a total picture of a phenomenon rather than considering parts in isolation.

It is suggested that qualitative research has six central traits (see Table 8.1) (Speziale and Carpenter, 2007).

Table 8.1 Six basic traits of qualitative research

Trait	Description
Belief in multiple realities	<ul><li>There is no one reality/truth</li><li>People actively construct their understanding of the world</li><li>People have different experiences of life</li><li>A number of perspectives are available in relation to any situation/phenomenon</li></ul>
An understanding of the nature of the phenomena being studies through appropriate methods is provided	<ul><li>There are multiple ways of understanding various phenomena</li><li>The most appropriate approach(es) to 'capturing' these understandings must be used</li><li>The phenomenon under consideration dictates the method to be used</li><li>Multiple forms of data collection are often used to ensure a full understanding of the research topic</li></ul>
Provides an understanding from the subject/participant's point of view	<ul><li>Qualitative research involves developing a theory in relation to a phenomenon – asking questions such as 'what do you experience of caring?' from someone with a learning disability</li></ul>
Research is conducted in the natural environment in which the phenomenon occurs	<ul><li>No attempt is made to control the environment</li><li>The natural environment provides a way of accessing the participant's perspective whilst in the 'space' that it occurs</li><li>Gives access to any cues or influences on the individual's perspective</li></ul>
The researcher as part of the process	<ul><li>Acceptance that all research is conducted in a subjective way</li><li>Researcher is seen as adding to the richness of the data</li></ul>
Data are said to be 'rich' and 'deep'	<ul><li>Data are collected in the form of words, describing the perspectives and experiences of the participants</li></ul>

Types of qualitative research

There a number of approaches to qualitative research, each with their own theoretical and philosophical underpinnings. The most common approaches are outlined below and an overview of their various aspects is presented in Table 8.2.

Phenomenology

This approach is based in a philosophical tradition developed by Edmund Husserl (1857–1938) and Martin Heidegger (1889–1976) which considers people's everyday experiences. The focus here is to explore the meaning that people attach to their lived experience and is closely related to **hermeneutics,** which centres on meaning and interpretation – how people interpret their experiences within a specific context. For example, if you wanted to know what it means to someone to be given a diagnosis of cancer, how they experience this, you might undertake a phenomenological study.

Grounded theory

Developed by sociologists Glaser and Strauss (1967), grounded theory is an approach originally forwarded as a way of developing theories and hypotheses that are 'grounded' in the data collected. Strauss and Corbin (1990) describe a grounded theory as one that 'is discovered, developed, and provisionally verified through systematic data collection and analysis of data pertaining to the phenomenon'. It is based on the idea that human behaviour is developed through people's interactions and their interpretation of these. It is often used to study social processes, considering the changes that occur over time in relation to particular experiences. In nursing it is frequently used to gain an understanding of the process through which people learn to manage and/or adapt to a new situation. For example, this approach could be used to consider how children adapt their lives over time following a diagnosis of diabetes.

Ethnography

This research approach has its roots in anthropology, being used to consider beliefs, values and shared meanings of people in particular cultures. Leininger (1985: 35) defined ethnography as 'the systematic process of observing, detailing, describing, documenting and analysing the lifeways or particular patterns of a culture (or subculture)'. Cultures in this context could relate to an entire social group (such as the culture of people from Romania) or to a small group (such as a particular ward

Table 8.2 Overview of qualitative research approaches

Approach	Types of research questions	Data collection	Example
Phenomenology	Meaning/lived experience	Unstructured interviews	Sin, J., Moone, N., Harris, P., Scully, E. & Wellman, N. (2012) 'Understanding the experiences and service needs of siblings of individuals with first-episode psychosis: a phenomenological study', *Early Intervention in Psychiatry*, 6: 53–59.
Grounded theory	Social settings Process questions	Interviews Observation	Lally, R.M., Hydeman, J.A., Henderson, H. & Edge, S.B. (2012) 'Exploring the first days of adjustment to cancer: a modification of acclimatising to breast cancer', *Cancer Nursing*, 35(1): 3–18.
Ethnography	Culture Beliefs and values	Participant observation Field notes Interviews	Bisholt, B.K.M. (2012) 'The learning process of recently graduated nurses in professional situations: experiences of an introduction program', *Nurse Education Today*, 32: 289–293.
Discourse analysis	Verbal interaction What power relationships are present in conversations?	Observation Recording of interactions Field notes	Fenwick, J., Burns, E., Sheehan, A. & Schmed, V. (2012) 'We only talk about breast feeding: a discourse analysis of infant feeding messages in antenatal group-based education', *Midwifery*, DOI: 10.1016/j.mid2012.02.006.
Action research	Implementing change	Mixed	Dengler, K.A., Wilson, V., Redshaw, S. & Scarfe, G. (2012) 'Appreciation of a child's journey: implementation of a cardiac action research project', *Nursing Research and Practice*, published online Article ID 145030.
Historical	Identifying historical roots and/or practices	Interviews Narratives Documentation	Oakes, P. (2012) 'Assessment of learning disabilities: a history', *Learning Disability Practice*, 15(1): 12–16.

setting). Therefore you could study the beliefs and values of people from Romania in relation to the care of people with learning disabilities. Alternatively, you could study how the culture of a particular residential home for people with learning disabilities impacts on the care given.

Action research

Action research can include both qualitative and quantitative approaches and is used to study the effects of actions when these are taken to change or improve something. There are various forms of action research, but the basic tenet is that it is a group activity (Speziale and Carpenter, 2007), usually involving some form of collaboration between the researcher and the participants – practitioners, patients or other stakeholders in the process – with a view to improving/changing practices in a specific area. It is also said to be context bound, in that the research is undertaken because of a defined issue related to a specific area. Its participants are seen as central to decision-making processes and have the final say as to whether changes are implemented or not. It is often seen as cyclic in nature with problems being identified, change made and impact evaluated. For instance you could use this approach to consider the most appropriate way to change how 'clinical handover' is organised in a particular ward setting.

Discourse Analysis

Discourse Analysis is relatively new to nursing research and looks at the ways in which people talk about particular issues, the systems people use in communicating with each other. It tries to uncover the rules that govern how people talk about things. Its basic premise is that language is not neutral: when talking, what is said and how it is said has particular meaning and intentions. Foucault's (1979) work has been particularly influential in this area, focusing on how power is exercised through the use of language. For example it would be possible to consider what power relations are present when qualified nurses talk to students and what values are present in the language they use.

Historical research

As a research approach, historical methods collect and interpret historical data in a systematic way. The aim is to provide new insights into a topic area not to summarise existing knowledge as might be done with a literature review (Speziale and Carpenter, 2007). Generally the form of historical research is underpinned by a particular theoretical framework, such as feminism or postmodernism. Historical research may be in the form of biographical accounts of individuals who provide oral histories of particular groups. For example oral histories could be taken from people who have experienced mental health institution at various points in the 20th century.

Activity

Find one piece of research for each of the research approaches identified in Table 8.2 relevant to your own field of nursing. Consider how each piece might inform your practice.

Critical appraisal

As discussed in relation to quantitative research, a number of tools are available to help you critically appraise research and many that are specifically aimed at qualitative research. Again, as identified in Chapter 6, guidelines for the reporting of research studies have been created by the EQUATOR network and these include qualitative studies guidance (see www.equator-network.org/home/). The most commonly recommended is COREQ (Consolidation Criteria for Reporting Qualitative Research). This is a checklist of 32 items aimed at research which uses interview or focus group approaches. This may be of help in identifying what should be included in qualitative research studies.

Activity

Locate the COREQ guidelines at www.equator-network.org and identify the aspects that are considered to be central to the designing and writing up of qualitative research.

Appendix 7 gives a generic approach to this form of critique, and those areas specific to qualitative research are highlighted and discussed below. The areas that are shared in both qualitative and quantitative research are discussed in Chapter 6. Again, as identified previously, having good research books to hand so you can check or clarify information as you go along is crucial to your success.

Activity

Find a critical appraisal tool for each of the research approaches identified in Table 8.2.

Research question and aims

Qualitative research normally will have a research question and not a hypothesis, as the intention is to generate understanding in relation to a phenomenon not to predict a relationship between variables. The research question can take two forms (Cormack, 1996):

1   Interrogative – namely, a statement phrased as a question, e.g. 'What is the lived experience of people admitted to hospital following a suicide attempt?'
2   Declarative – namely, a statement which 'declares' the purpose of the study, e.g. 'It is intended to study the experience of people admitted to hospital following a suicide attempt.'

The best research questions are short and clearly identify a specific area of study. The question should set the scene for the research design that will allow the question to be answered. Some researchers will pose a series of questions, others identify a series of aims in relation to the question asked. The research question and aims should have the same intentions.

Literature review

An extensive literature review is not always the starting point of qualitative research. Often only sufficient literature to provide a focus for the study will be considered. In phenomenological research the literature may not be reviewed until after the data have been collected and analysed. In grounded theory the literature is reviewed at various points throughout the data collection process and is used as a comparison for the interim research findings. This lack of initial literature review is to ensure that the analysis of the data is not influenced by what is already known about the topic. However, there is an expectation that the findings will be considered in light of the available literature, so that the study can be compared with other work and any issues regarding the transferability of findings to other settings can be identified.

Where a literature review is provided, the criteria identified by Parahoo (2006) described in Chapter 6 (p. 80) can be applied.

Methodology

The chosen methodology should enable the research question to be answered. If the question asks about the meaning of something or an individual's experience, then you would expect to see a phenomenological design. If the stated aim is to investigate issues related to culture – beliefs, values, social norms – then an ethnographic approach would be more appropriate. There should be a match between what the researcher wants to know and the methodology used to answer the question. Table 8.2

gives an idea of the methodologies expected to be seen in relation to particular areas of study.

Reflexivity

Whilst researcher involvement in the research process is a central tenet of qualitative research, there is also an expectation that researchers will discuss their beliefs, values, ideas and personal biases relating to the topic they are exploring and this is usually given in the form of a reflective account. This reflexivity is seen as having two purposes. First it makes the investigators aware of how their own beliefs may influence the data collection and interpretation. Having explored their own perspectives it is normally expected that researchers will put aside their beliefs in what is termed as **bracketing**. Here researchers are expected not to make judgements about the appropriateness of what they see or hear, instead being open to what the data reveal rather than imposing their own beliefs on it. The second aspect relates to acknowledging that the researcher is part of the research process and ensures that the reader is aware of this.

Activity

Identify an area you would be interested in researching. Write a short reflective piece identifying what beliefs and values you have in relation to the area and how that might impact on any research you undertook.

However, whilst this process is an integral part of qualitative research, often the reflective account is missing from published work. The word limits imposed by journal publishers on authors of papers frequently result in this aspect being left out. When this is the case, the only insight given into the researchers' perspectives and backgrounds in terms of the research phenomenon is gained through examining their qualifications and job titles given at the beginning of the article.

Ethical issues

As identified in Chapter 6, all health service research requires ethical approval, however the nature of qualitative research brings a distinct set of ethical issues into view. The interpersonal nature of most qualitative research (i.e. that the researcher and participants are in direct contact and form a close, albeit brief, trusting relationship) requires the researcher to be aware of any possible emotional impact the research may have on participants. Speziale and Carpenter (2007) identify various aspects that are important in qualitative research, and these are areas you should consider when doing a critical appraisal:

1 Informed consent – within qualitative research participants must be allowed to withdraw this consent at any point. 'Process informed' consent is often adopted, where a participant's consent will be re-evaluated at various points within the study and involvement stopped if required.

2 Confidentiality and anonymity – the one-to-one interaction between participant and researcher means that anonymity is not possible in the same way as in quantitative research; the researcher will obviously know where the data came from. However confidentiality can and must be maintained with every effort made to ensure that participants are not recognisable in the data used to support descriptions of results.

3 The researcher–participant relationship – the researcher must be clear about the boundaries of this relationship. This is a particular issue for healthcare professionals, who may find their role as care provider conflicting with their role of researcher.

4 Sensitive issues – some of the issues discussed during data collection can be distressing for the participants and/or the researcher. It is important that the researcher identifies mechanisms for dealing with such issues and how participants will be supported following data collection.

Activity

Imagine you are conducting a research study discussing a topic which may cause the participants to become distressed. What support do you think it would be important to offer to the participants?

Sampling/participant selection

Individuals are usually selected to participate in particular research because they will have had experience of or are involved in the phenomenon being studied. For instance, if the research question is 'What is the lived experience of people with schizophrenia?' people selected to participate in the study would be people with schizophrenia, as only they would be able to describe their experiences.

As the intention with qualitative research is to gain a greater understanding of the area of interest, not to generalise findings, randomised sampling is not an issue here. There are various approaches to sampling the population of interest:

- convenience – the most conveniently available people are selected, those who are closest to hand and relevant to the phenomenon of interest;
- snowballing – a form of convenience sampling where having identified an informant to tell you about the phenomenon, they then identify someone else;

- purposive or purposeful – selecting people who can tell you about the research phenomenon; this approach tends to be used in phenomenological studies;
- theoretical – a framework is created in which the principal concepts related to the study are identified and individuals are selected to participate who are judged to have theoretical purpose/relevance; the researcher clearly states the basic types of participants to be included and how these individuals will facilitate the collection of appropriate data to describe the phenomenon. This approach is most often seen in grounded theory.

Sample sizes in qualitative research are normally small in comparison to quantitative research. It is not unusual to see research conducted on just 10 people. The nature of the data collected and subsequent analysis makes large samples almost impossible to handle. For example, one 45-minute interview can produce 30 pages of transcribed information. If you have just 10 participants this results in 300 pages requiring analysis. The aim of qualitative research is to reduce this huge amount of information to a manageable size without losing the participants' intended meaning.

The sample size is largely decided by the type of research, the quality of the information provided by the participants and the sampling approach used. Often qualitative researchers talk about reaching **data saturation**, particularly in grounded theory. This is the point where no new information is being collected from participants and is usually the point where data collection stops. So, for example, if data saturation is reached after interviewing 12 people then no further interviews will be conducted.

Data collection

There are various forms of data collection available to the qualitative researcher, but all of them involve the collection of 'words' in some shape or form. Table 8.3 provides an overview of the main types of activity. In appraising a study it is important to consider whether the form of data collection used will provide the researcher with the most appropriate data.

It is essential that a study identifies how the information from participants was recorded. Many researchers will use audio recording devices, some may incorporate video recording, to ensure that non-verbal responses are captured. Whilst field notes are useful and add to the picture, they tend to be incomplete and do not enable the researcher to revisit the interaction in its original form.

Data analysis

Polit and Beck (2008) propose that qualitative data analysis is more difficult to do than quantitative analysis but easier to understand, which is a bonus for those who are critiquing rather than doing the research. However, it is not always easy to fully appraise the findings as you cannot know if the authors have given an appropriate representation of participants' narratives.

Table 8.3 Types of data collection

Type	Description
Interviews	• Unstructured – no prepared questions apart from asking them to talk about the phenomenon of interest • Semi-structured – a guide asking open questions related to the areas of interest, prepared in advance • (Structure – not used in qualitative research)
Focus groups	• Group interviews, 6–12 people discussing a topic
Observation	• Participant observation – the researcher is part of the group and is involved in its activities • Observer–participant – the researcher generally observes and may interview members of the group and may also participate in some activities • Complete observer – no interaction between observer and participant
Field notes	• In ethnography these involve documenting of observations, narratives • In phenomenology these may involve recording of individual expressions and other aspects not captured by audio recording of interviews
Diaries	• Unstructured – where people are asked simply to record their thoughts and feelings • Structured – where people are asked to write about specific aspects
Documentation	• Patient notes, historical records, health service documentation and records; published and unpublished works

All qualitative analysis involves some sort of content analysis where researchers create categories and themes from the data. As these categories are created, a coding system is then developed which allows statements made by participants to be grouped together in particular categories. Once such categories have been identified these may then be further grouped into themes. Data can be handled manually or analysed using computer-assisted qualitative data analysis systems (CAQDAS) such as such as ATLAS.ti and NVivo. However, as there are a number of approaches to qualitative research, the content analysis takes various forms. Note this lack of a universal approach can make it difficult for you to critically appraise the work.

When critically appraising a qualitative analysis you are looking to see whether the author has given you enough information to make a judgement as to whether the analysis has been conducted in an appropriate way. There are a number of basic tenets you would expect to be described:

1   Data transcription – how the data are translated from audio to a written form; what steps were taken to ensure data were of the best quality, including identification of problems related to transcription (e.g. background noise, poor tape quality, participant's voice inaudible).
2   Identification of tool used for analysis – a number of tools would be available and the one chosen should be appropriate to the research methodology. For example you

would not expect a grounded theory methodology to include Colaizzi's (1978) approach which is specific to phenomenology. The researcher involved should clearly identify the approach taken and you should be able to follow this step-by-step through the paper.

3 Interpretation – this occurs at the same time as the analysis as the researcher reads and re-reads the data and the codes, categories/themes and tries to make sense of the data. The writer should give details of how the interpretation was arrived at.

Activity

Find three different examples of tools that can be used in the analysis of qualitative data.

Issues of rigour

As Speziale and Carpenter (2007: 48) have pointed out, decisions as to the rigour of a particular research study is a 'judgement call'. They go on to suggest that two fundamental characteristics of qualitative research should be present when making this judgement as to whether it meets the implicit goal of providing an accurate account of participants' perspective:

1 Is there adequate attention to the collection of information?
2 Is there confirmation of the accuracy of the information?

Table 8.4   Criteria for assessing rigour of qualitative research

Criteria	Ways of identifying if criteria are met
Credibility	• Findings returned to participants for confirmation that they are a true representation of their experiences • All data are accounted for, including instances where the data are inconsistent with other findings • Triangulation
Dependability	• Reporting of unexpected events and how dealt with • Recording methods ensured quality of data • Triangulation
Confirmability	• Evidence of reflexivity • Provision of an 'audit trail' to enable the thought and decision-making processes to be identified (a research diary or recording mechanisms within CAQDAS)
Transferability	• Providing a full description of the research setting and participants • Identifying that the findings have relevance to similar situations • Theoretical triangulation
Authenticity	• The reality of the participants' lives is conveyed, enabling you to understand the range of feelings experienced by those involved

An alternative way for considering the rigour of qualitative research is provided by Lincoln and Guba (1985) and Guba and Lincoln (1994). Table 8.4 provides an overview of the proposed criteria.

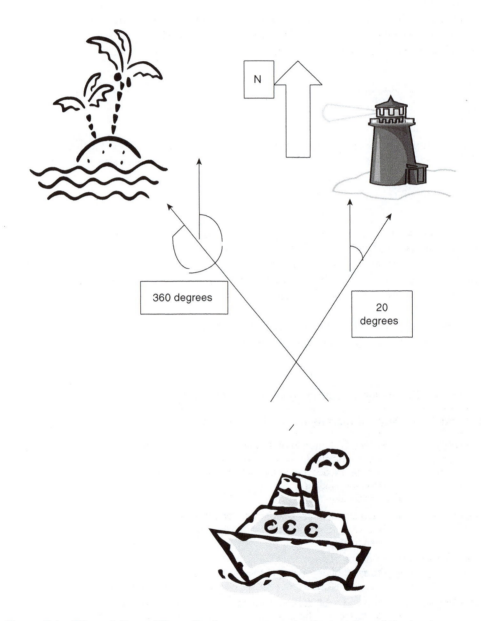

Figure 8.1   Triangulation – Where the lines cross marks the location of the boat

Triangulation is a strategy used in qualitative research to ensure that the approach has rigour and increases the credibility of results. The idea comes from a navigation term used to describe how sailors or pilots plot the location of their ship/ plane. Imagine you are on a boat in the middle of the ocean, you know the location of the lighthouse in the distance and an island to the west. Using a compass you take bearing readings (the angle between the lighthouse and north on the compass, and the island and the north point) and find these to be 20 degrees and 360 degrees respectively. You plot each line on a map and if the readings are correct, the lines should intersect at a certain point identifying your position (Figure 8.1).

Triangulation in qualitative research is based on the idea that the phenomenon of interest can be 'plotted' from different angles so a clearer description of it is given. Four types of triangulation are possible (Denzin, 1989):

1   Data triangulation – where more than one source of data is collected. This can be done in three ways:

  i   Time – collecting data at different points in time: for instance you might interview people at intervals of three, six and twelve months in relation to a particular phenomenon.
  ii   Space – collecting data from different sites; perhaps including different inpatient units in a study.
  iii   Person – collecting information from different groups of people: for example, interviewing nurses on band 5, 6 and 7; or service users and their carers.

2   Methodological triangulation – two or more research methods are used in:

  i   The research design – for example, combining qualitative and quantitative approaches.
  ii   The data collection techniques – for example using diaries and interviews.

3   Investigator triangulation – here two or more investigators, each having their own specific area of expertise, will collect, analyse and interpret the data.
4   Theoretical triangulation – having more than one theory underpinning the analysis of the data. As the data are analysed it is viewed through the 'lens' of different theories to see if alternative interpretations arise from examining it in multiple ways.

EBP Activity

Choose one of the research articles identified in Table 8.2 and critically appraise it using the questions in Appendix 7. Identify the aspects/questions where you need to develop further skills and knowledge. Develop an action plan outlining how you will develop the knowledge and skills you require to complete the task appropriately.

Summary

- There are a number of approaches to qualitative research, each with their own theoretical and philosophical underpinning, generally focusing on how people describe their experiences, perspectives, understanding and beliefs/values.
- Ethical issues take a particular form in qualitative research.
- Sample sizes in qualitative research are normally small in comparison to quantitative research. Individuals are usually selected to participate in particular research because they have experience or are involved in the phenomenon being studied.
- There are various forms of data collection available to the qualitative researcher, but most of them involve the collecting of 'words' in some shape or form and analysis involves some sort of content analysis where the researcher creates categories and themes from the data.

Further reading

Polit, D.F. and Beck, C.T. (2008) *Nursing Research: Generating and Assessing Evidence for Nursing Practice* (8th edn). Philadelphia: Lippincott Williams and Wilkins. Gives a good introduction to the various aspects of qualitative research and its approaches.

Speziale, H.J.S. and Carpenter, D.R. (2007) *Qualitative Research in Nursing* (4th edn). Philadelphia: Lippincott Williams and Wilkins. Provides an overview of various aspects of qualitative research, the different approaches and guidelines to help in the critical appraisal of the different methods.

E-resources

Critical Appraisal Skills Programme: provides a range of resources to help with developing the skills associated with EBP. Also provides a range of critical appraisal tools. www.casp-uk.net

Qual Page: provides resources and information related to qualitative research. The methods section provides an overview of different qualitative methodologies. www. qualitativeresearch.uga.ed/QualPage/methods.html

Netting the Evidence Google Search Engine: searches 107 sites associated with EBP. http://tinyurl.com/2poh3a

9

Systematic Reviews and Evidence-Based Practice

Learning Outcomes

By the end of the chapter you will be able to:

- discuss the systematic review process and its basic traits;
- identify key areas for consideration when critically appraising systematic reviews;
- identify issues to be considered when assessing the rigour of systematic reviews.

Introduction

The explosion of literature related to healthcare has made it almost impossible for any practitioner to keep abreast with all current research findings. It is suggested that the information relating to biomedicine doubles every 20 years (Davies, 2011). David Sackett (2008) stated that to keep up-to-date in his speciality he would need to read at least 17 papers a day, every day of the year. **Systematic reviews** (SRs) provide a rigorous review of research findings in relation to a specific question, saving practitioners the time and effort it would take to search and appraise a large body of evidence. Whilst it is not expected that health professionals in general undertake SRs (they can be both complex and time consuming to complete) there is a need to be able to appraise them and evaluate the usefulness of the findings for practice.

Pearson et al. (2007) see systematic reviews as fundamental to EBP, providing practitioners with sound evidence on which to base practice. SR is often a term that is used interchangeably with **meta-analysis**, but as you will see from the discussion below the two are not the same, the latter can be part of the former but is not always present. SRs have been primarily associated with quantitative research, but increasingly systematic reviews of qualitative research are being undertaken with an accompanying **meta-synthesis** of the qualitative findings. There are some SRs which consider both qualitative and quantitative studies and provide both a meta-analysis and meta-synthesis of relevant studies. As SRs provide an overview of primary research they can be of immense use in clinical practice.

The processes in a systematic review can seem a little overwhelming to the novice appraiser, however if considered step-by-step it is possible to gain a picture of whether a review is applicable to your own area of practice. This chapter will consider the methods and approaches used in SRs and the areas to be considered when critically appraising this form of evidence.

What is a systematic review?

As identified in Chapter 1 in many ways EBP is seen as having its origins in Professor Archie Cochrane's criticisms of the medical profession for its failure to use the body of evidence available to them in an appropriate way. Prior to the emergence of EBP, summaries of studies more frequently appeared in the form of what Greenhalgh (2006) terms as 'journalistic reviews'. Here papers were reviewed, selected and analysed in an ad hoc manner, subject to the vagaries of the person conducting the literature review. In many ways this left any interpretation provided open to accusations of bias, and the lack of a systematic approach gives the reader little evidence on which to consider the credibility of the findings. However, since the advent of EBP, SRs have become more prevalent, generally conducted using rigorous designs, often adhering to a standard format or at the very least one that is made explicit and is reproducible. For example to improve the reporting of systematic reviews and meta-analyses, the EQUATOR network (see Chapter 6) provides guidelines known as PRISMA (Preferred Reporting Items for Systematic Reviews and Meta-Analyses) which identify what should be included and considered when designing and writing up meta-analyses. Many meta-analyses now follow the structure provided by the PRISMA statement.

Activity

Visit the PRISMA website (www.prisma-statement.org/). Identify two of the items on the checklist provided in relation to a meta-analysis that you feel you know least about. Draw up and implement an action plan to develop your learning in relation to the two aspects.

Systematic reviews are a form of research, often termed as **secondary research** as secondary sources of data are used, usually coming from primary research that has collected data from original sources (participants, subjects, etc.). As the Cochrane Collaboration (2012) identifies, SRs 'seek to collate all evidence that fits pre-specified eligibility criteria in order to address a specific research question'. The process of 'collating' this evidence is a systematic process – Box 9.1 identifies the steps associated with SRs. Pearson et al. (2007) have added a further step which involves the creation of a best practice guide based on the evidence identified in the systematic review. As you can see they are very similar to the steps identified in relation to EBP.

Box 9.1 Systematic review process

- Formulate question, aim, outcomes.

- Define terms.
- Identify inclusion/exclusion criteria.
- Identify search strategy.
- Search the literature.
- Appraise the evidence.
- Synthesise the data where appropriate or provide a narrative account of findings.
- Conclude and make recommendation.

Types of systematic reviews

There are two main types of SRs – qualitative and quantitative. The basic steps of each are the same; however differences occur in the data extraction and summarising. Whilst in both types of SR the reviewer is 'pooling' the results from 'like' studies and creating a larger data set for analysis (Pearson et al., 2007), the underpinning philosophies and methods used are different. The pooling of quantitative data is seen as an aggregating of the findings, the pooling of qualitative findings can be an aggregation or interpretation of findings depending on the approach used. A meta-analysis can also be seen as giving a picture of the effectiveness of an intervention, while meta-synthesis increases understanding of a phenomenon of interest. Where statistical data are the focus a meta-analysis is conducted. If the data are qualitative in nature than a meta-synthesis is undertaken. A number of tools are readily available to assist in these processes (see Box 9.2).

Box 9.2 Electronic tools for data extraction and synthesis

Review Manager	Commonly know as 'rev-man', created by Cochrane Collaboration for systematic reviews of effectiveness studies.
Systems for the Unified Management of the Assessment and Review of Information (SUMARI)	Created by Joanna Briggs Institute this is a collection of tools to enable the systematic review of various types of evidence: • MAStAri – effectiveness studies; • ACTURI – economic studies; • QARI – qualitative studies; • NOTARI – text, expert opinion and discourses.

Meta-analysis is defined by Greenhalgh (2006: 122) as 'a statistical synthesis of the numerical results of several trials which all address the same question'. It enables the bringing together of results for studies that are said to homogeneous in nature – considering the same outcome of the same intervention, on the same population – in an objective way. The power to detect relationships between variables is increased due to the increased sample size created through combining studies. This in turn allows conclusions to be drawn about the size of the effect of an intervention.

Meta-synthesis is a growing area of interest; however it is not without its dissenters. There is heated debate around whether meta-synthesis of qualitative findings is appropriate or indeed possible. For those that advocate meta-synthesis, some would propose that only findings from studies using the same methodology (phenomenology, ethnography, etc.) are possible, whilst others would argue that it is possible and appropriate to combine findings from various methodologies. Polit and Beck (2008) identify three approaches to meta-synthesis – Noblit and Hare's; Paterson, Thorne, Can and Joilling's; and Sandelowski and Barroso's. The main aspects of these are identified in Table 9.1.

Table 9.1 Meta-synthesis approaches

Approach	Description	Example
Noblit & Hare (1988) (Meta-ethnography)	• Considers how studies relate to each other (either seen as being reciprocal – comparable; or refutational – in opposition) • Translating studies, ensuring main concepts are reflected • Synthesising the various translations into comprehensible whole • Providing a narrative account of the synthesis	Ring, N., Jepson, R., Hoskins, G., Wilson, C., Pinnock, H., Sheikh, A. & Wyke, S. (2011) 'Understanding what helps or hinders asthma action plan use: a systematic review and synthesis of the qualitative research', *Patient Education and Counseling*, 85: e131–e143
Paterson et al. (2001)	Three components: • Meta-data analysis – analysis of the finding • Meta-method – the rigour with which each study is conducted is incorporated into the meta-synthesis • Meta-theory – the study's theoretical underpinnings are analysed • These three components are brought together to produce a meta-synthesis of findings	Price, S.J. (2009) 'Becoming a nurse: a meta-study of early professional socialisation and career choice in nursing', *Journal of Advanced Nursing*, 65(1): 11–19.
Sandelowski & Barroso (2006)	• An integration of findings • Integrating interpretation into a new description of the phenomenon of interest	Taverner, T., Closs, J. & Briggs, M. (2011) 'A meta-synthesis of research on leg ulceration and neuropathic pain', *British Journal of Nursing*, 20 (supplement): 18–27.

The generalisability of qualitative meta-syntheses is also hotly debated. As qualitative research itself makes no claims of generalisability, with the emphasis being seen as providing thick description and providing insight into phenomena, there are concerns about making such claims in relation to meta-synthesis of results. Nevertheless, the pulling together of 'like' studies and providing wider consideration of a particular phenomenon in relation to a particular group can have practical uses.

Critiquing a systematic review

As identified in Chapter 6 there are a number of tools available to help you perform a critical appraisal (Appendix 8 gives a generic approach to particular areas to be addressed in critically appraising systematic reviews). As always, when critically appraising it is helpful to have good research books to hand so you can check or clarify information as you go along.

Activity

Find a tool suitable for critically appraising a meta-analysis and one for a meta-synthesis.

Question, objectives and inclusion criteria

All systematic reviews should have a clearly identifiable question generally present in the PICO format or a variation of this. Without this the reviewer and the reader will not be able to decide what are relevant papers to be included and what should be rejected. Whilst a particular question such as 'Does eating breakfast improve cognitive functioning in children?' may initially sound appropriate, when you start to pull it apart and consider each aspect, such as what is meant by children (all under-18s or a specific group?), breakfast (a slice of toast or a 'full English'?) and cognitive functioning (alertness, memory, understanding, completion of tests?), then it becomes apparent that the need for clear identification of the various facets is central to the whole process.

As with any research the objectives should be clearly stated and flow from the question. The inclusion criteria identify the limits of the review and give a clear indication of what is to be included in the review and what is not. Sound justifications are expected to be present for the setting of the limits as well as a clear exploration of the implications of these for the review.

Searching for the literature

The methodology used to identify the literature relevant to a particular SR is a central issue when judging the rigour of a SR. As Pearson et al. (2007) have pointed out, the quality of the SR is reduced if the search strategy is poorly designed and implemented. In undertaking a review, a reviewer must be sure that all studies relevant to a topic are identified. This often requires a complex search strategy in which search terms are clearly identified, thus ensuring that any literature relevant to the review is located. The same principles as discussed in Chapter 5 apply in identifying what terms are appropriate.

In searching the literature it is expected that:

- all relevant electronic databases are included;
- the hand searching of printed journals is undertaken;
- reference lists are checked for potential sources;
- grey literature is considered;
- raw data and other unpublished sources generated through personal communications are included where appropriate.

In critically appraising a SR it is important to consider if all relevant sources of literature have been included as this may have an impact on the rigour of the review.

Activity

List databases and other sources of information you would consider key to finding literature related to your own area of practice.

Quality assessment

The quality of the evidence to be included in the review will generally be assessed and some form of critical appraisal of each study will be undertaken. Therefore the tool used for this appraisal should be identified and be appropriate to the type of research under consideration. In undertaking this appraisal, the Cochrane Collaboration advocates the weighting of those studies included in terms of strength – the stronger the study, the greater weight it is given in the meta-analysis. The Joanna Briggs Institute advocates rejecting those studies identified as not being of an appropriate standard.

The use of two critical appraisers is the norm in SRs. The appraisers act independently, subjecting each piece of evidence for inclusion in the SR to a robust appraisal process. The two then confer and reach an agreement as to the quality of each individual study for inclusion in the review.

Data extraction

The form of data extraction should be clearly identified. Various tools are available to assist with the extraction of data (see Box 9.2). For quantitative reviews, initial information should be apparent in relation to the studies and is usually presented in the form of tables identifying:

- each study's inclusion criteria;
- sample base and drop-out rates;
- patient characteristics, e.g. age, gender, ethnicity;
- the intervention – details of the exact form of intervention and how it was delivered (e.g. routes, dosages, timing, instructions for delivery);
- the outcome measures – the reviewer should clearly identify what outcome measures are under consideration;
- results.

In relation to qualitative reviews it is expected that the study's methodology (phenomenology, ethnography, etc.), cultural features (age, socioeconomic group and ethnicity) and form of data collection (interview, focus group, etc.) will be clearly highlighted.

These tables will allow you to compare various studies and help you to make a judgement as to the rigour of the SR. If a table indicates there is significant heterogeneity within the studies then it is unlikely that the results of the study will be subjected to meta-analysis. It is possible to conduct a meta-synthesis of heterogeneous qualitative studies and this is discussed later in the chapter.

Summarising the evidence

It is not always possible or appropriate to pool data in the form of a meta-analysis and in such cases a narrative integration, a written summary of findings, is provided. The narrative should be clear, concise and give a clear description data.

Activity

Locate the following article – Alagiakrishnan, K., Bhanji, R.S. and Kurian, M. (2012) 'Evaluation and management of oropharyngeal dysphagia in different types of dementia: a systematic review', *Archives of Gerontology and Geriatrics*. http://dxdoiorg/10.1016/j.archger.2012.04.011 – which provides a narrative summary of the findings. If there are aspects of the information which you do not have sufficient knowledge to appraise, create an action plan identifying how you will develop this knowledge.

Meta-analysis

Greenhalgh (2006) has suggested that the mere term strikes fear into the hearts of many students and practitioners, being seen as a statistical analysis of statistical analyses. However, as Greenhalgh advocates, often the meta-analysis is easier to understand than the original statistics. Akobeng (2005) proposed that the meta-analysis has two parts:

1   Calculating a measure of treatment effect (common measures are odds ratios, relative risk and risk differences – see Table 9.2) and confidence interval for each study.
2   Calculating the overall treatment effect.

Table 9.2   Treatment effect measures

Measure	Description
Odds ratio	Measures ratio of the odds of an outcome in the intervention group to the odds of the outcome in the control group 1 = no difference between groups Undesirable outcomes; less than 1 = intervention effective in reducing risk
Relative risk (RR)	Measures the ratio of risk in the intervention group to that in the control group RR of 1.0 = no difference between the groups
Risk difference (RD)	The absolute difference in the outcome rate in the groups RD of 0 = no difference between groups
Absolute risk reduction (ARR)	The difference in event rates between the control group and the treatment group
Numbers needed to treat (NNT)	The number of people who need to be treated to prevent one undesirable outcome

The reviewer begins by deciding which of the outcome measures of the studies reviewed are to be used for the meta-analysis – in most studies a number of outcomes are measured, although only some of these may be of interest to the reviewer. The findings in relation to these outcomes are presented as treatment effect measures which identify the strength and direction of the relationship between the independent and dependent variables.

The reviewers will also identify what is known as statistical heterogeneity – that is, how diverse the effects are across the various studies. This is usually demonstrated through the use of forest plot graphs – sometimes referred to as 'blobbograms' (see Figure 9.1 for an example). Each horizontal line is the confidence interval for an individual study. The symbol or 'blob' in the middle of each line is the estimated treatment effect of the study (odds ratio, relative risk, etc.), the size of the blob represents the size of the effect. The width of the line represents the 95 per cent confidence interval of this treatment effect – as identified in Chapter 7, the wider the interval the less precise the estimate. The black line down the middle is the 'line of no effect'. In this example if the confidence interval of a particular study crosses the 'line of no effect' it means either there is no significant difference between treatment groups and/ or the sample is too small to be confident that that there is an effect. The heterogeneity of studies can be instantly assessed in forest plot graphs as the more scattered the lines the more heterogeneous the results. The more heterogeneous the results, the less confidence there is in the ability to use the results in practice.

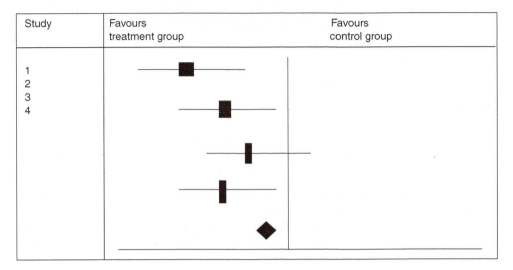

Figure 9.1   Forest plot graphs

The diamond below all the horizontal lines represents the pooled effect of the data. Where this is placed reflects whether overall there is confidence that one treatment is better than the other. On the line means that for the average person there is little choice between the two, while to the left of the line identifies one is better than the other.

If the studies are seen as homogeneous and heterogeneity of treatment effects are identified between studies, Khan et al. (2003) suggest that this may be due to differences in the characteristics of:

- the population;
- interventions;
- outcomes;
- study design.

For example, if in one study the sample of older people included the 'young old' (between the ages of 65 and 80 years) and in another the sample was made up of 'old older' people (80 years old +) that would represent a heterogeneous population and would explain why differences in the effect of an intervention were seen. Where none of the above is apparent, Khan et al. suggest that heterogeneity may be a result of **publication bias**. This type of bias occurs due to a tendency in some areas for only positive results to be published, and in using such findings for SRs a bias towards effectiveness is likely. It is expected that the reviewers will explore this possibility.

Frequently in meta-analysis it can be identified that where a number of trials have reported no significance, the pooled data will result in statistical significance. The

Cochrane Collaboration logo is a representation of the most famous incidence of this pooling which identified significance. It represents a meta-analysis of seven RCTs related to the effect of steroids on women expected to give birth prematurely. Only two of the seven trials showed statistical significance in terms of improving the survival of the child, however the meta-analysis showed that in mothers who received steroids, their infants were 30–50 per cent less likely to die.

Activity

Visit the Cochrane website at www.cochrane.org/ and view the logo.

A sensitivity analysis is usually undertaken to identify any changes in the original data that may have occurred as a result of pooling. This involves re-analysing data from different perspectives to see if this has an impact on the results. If substantial changes are reported to have occurred as a result of pooling data then caution should be taken in applying the results to your own area of practice.

Activity

Visit the Cochrane Library at www.thecochranelibrary.com/view/0/index.html and access a meta-analysis relevant to your own area of practice and familiarise yourself with the organisation and layout of a systematic review.

Meta-synthesis

Meta-synthesis is derived from the Greek words *meta* meaning 'change, alteration transcend or going beyond' and *synthesis* meaning 'to put together' (Collins Dictionary, 1998), which suggest this is about putting together things in a way that goes beyond the features of the individual items. Finlayson and Dixon (2008) have suggested it is the bringing together of the findings of qualitative research in an effort to provide a clearer picture of the phenomenon of interest. Evans and Pearson (2001) also identified that a meta-synthesis allows systematic and critical examination/interpretation.

There are a variety of approaches to meta-synthesis, indeed as Pope et al. (2007) identified, various terms are used to describe the processes (such as interpretive synthesis, meta-study, qualitative meta-analysis). However, Pearson et al. (2007) claim these approaches generally involve:

- data extraction – identifying the research findings in the form of metaphors, themes, categories and/or concepts present within the study;
- data synthesis – grouping the findings into categories;
- grouping the categories into synthesised findings.

The processes involved are very similar to that of primary qualitative research, and as in any form of qualitative research the reviewers are providing an interpretation of the findings. The process appears on the face of it to be a simple one, but in reality is quite complex and requires a rigorous examination of the studies. The aim is to provide an accurate representation of the findings which gives a full picture of the essential characteristics of the phenomenon under consideration. The specific approach used to achieve this is expected to be clearly outlined to enable you to judge the rigour of the process and the appropriateness of the review for application within your own area of practice.

Whereas heterogeneity is an issue of great concern within meta-analysis this is less so within meta-synthesis (Evans and Pearson, 2001). In qualitative research heterogeneity is anticipated; the issue for reviewers is to ensure that differences are acknowledged, compared across studies and accounted for within the new interpretation.

Conclusions, recommendations/limitations

The reviewers should justify their conclusions and recommendations in relation both to their application to practice and the implications for healthcare. Recommendations in terms of future research agendas are normally included. Other information such as costs involved in treatment regimes should be addressed.

Applicability to practice

The criteria identified in Chapter 6 for judging applicability to practice are equally valid for SRs, however there is also a specific aspect that should be considered. The specificity of the systematic review question means that a very narrow aspect of care is being considered and there is a clear need to place this within the 'bigger picture' of the care environment you are concerned with. You need to consider whether factors not considered in the review will have implications for applying the results to your own area of practice.

EBP Activity

Identify a SR specific to your area of practice and critically appraise it using the criteria identified in Appendix 8.

Summary

- SRs provide a rigorous review of research findings in relation to a specific question and as such they are fundamental to EBP, providing practitioners with sound evidence on which to base practice.
- The SR review process involves the 'pooling' of results from 'like' studies and creating a larger data set for analysis. This is known as meta-analysis in relation to quantitative research and meta-synthesis with regard to qualitative findings.
- If there is significant heterogeneity within the studies reviewed in a SR it is unlikely that the results of the study will be subjected to meta-analysis.
- There are a variety of approaches to meta-synthesis; it is important that a clear description of the approach is provided to allow you to make decisions as to the rigour of the review.

Further reading

Akobeng, A.K. (2005) 'Understanding systematic reviews and meta-analysis'; www.adc.bmj. com (Accessed August 2008). Gives a good introduction to meta-analysis.

Finlayson, K. and Dixon, A. (2008) 'Qualitative meta-synthesis: a guide for the novice', *Nurse Researcher*, 15(2): 59–71. Explores the central themes of this approach.

Greenhalgh, T. (2006) *How to Read a Paper: The Basics of Evidence-Based Medicine* (3rd edn). Oxford: Blackwell. Provides guidelines for and a clear description of how to critique meta-analysis.

E-resources

CETL Reusable Learning Objects: this website provides reusable learning objects (RLOs) related to a range of topics. These are multimedia overviews of various topics. The 'EBP' section contains an RLO related to systematic reviews. www.rlo-cetl.ac.uk/index.php

Campbell Collaboration: prepares, promotes and updates systematic reviews of social interventions. www.campbellcollaboration.org

Centre for Reviews and Dissemination: has systematic reviews on selected topics, a database of reviews and resources for the conducting of systematic reviews. www.york.ac.uk/inst/crd

Cochrane Collaboration: promotes, supports and prepares systematic reviews, mainly in relation to effectiveness. www.cochrane.org/

Joanna Briggs Institute: promotes evidence-based healthcare through systematic reviews and a range of resources aimed at promoting evidence synthesis, transfer and utilisation. www. joannabriggs.edu.au

Conclusion to Part 2

The aim of Part 2 was to provide you with the necessary skills, knowledge and tools to enable you to critically appraise a range of evidence. Hopefully you have now:

- identified a number of papers relevant to your own area of practice;
- found a number of appropriate tools to aid you in your critical appraisal;
- identified gaps in your knowledge and developed action plans to allow you to fill in the gaps;
- developed confidence in your ability to critically appraise evidence in an appropriate way.

Part 2 ends with a word search puzzle in which there are 21 words associated with Chapters 6, 7, 8 and 9. What are they? The answers can be found on p. 178.

J	T	R	I	A	L	U	O	U	T	Q	T	V	Q	U	X	T	E	V	X
A	G	M	U	Q	V	A	R	I	A	B	L	E	S	E	L	R	O	E	D
S	K	S	Q	Q	L	X	R	I	G	O	U	R	E	B	H	U	M	G	H
K	V	S	J	R	S	J	C	F	D	N	B	T	Y	T	N	S	N	Z	S
K	W	Y	B	F	N	K	O	Q	A	P	F	B	E	R	Z	T	J	R	T
M	A	Z	R	T	O	Q	N	N	Z	R	E	J	U	A	Z	W	D	A	R
O	V	H	A	T	W	E	F	Z	R	O	Z	F	I	N	Y	O	E	N	A
D	S	Y	C	D	B	Y	I	X	E	B	U	F	J	S	H	R	P	D	T
E	M	P	K	W	A	R	R	K	L	A	P	E	Q	F	F	T	E	O	I
R	E	O	E	A	L	E	M	E	I	B	T	T	L	E	F	H	N	M	F
Y	T	T	T	J	L	D	A	F	A	I	K	I	A	R	E	I	D	I	I
A	A	H	I	L	R	V	B	X	B	L	D	C	L	A	W	N	A	S	E
K	A	E	N	D	E	O	I	G	I	I	G	D	N	B	Z	E	B	E	D
E	N	S	G	I	Q	B	L	E	L	T	U	U	L	I	W	S	I	D	S
U	A	I	T	U	R	K	I	E	I	Y	F	G	K	L	Z	S	L	O	S
N	L	S	T	V	P	B	T	Z	T	F	F	Z	U	I	V	E	I	A	B
K	Y	C	W	R	W	J	Y	A	Y	M	E	A	N	T	K	R	T	C	P
L	S	U	J	E	M	I	C	B	A	S	N	K	M	Y	V	W	Y	G	O
S	I	U	F	R	T	Z	Y	P	R	I	V	A	L	I	D	I	T	Y	T
C	S	K	C	R	E	D	I	B	I	L	I	T	Y	T	D	F	R	C	B

Part 3

Making Changes

10

Moving from Evidence to Practice Development

Learning Outcomes

By the end of the chapter you will be able to:

- identify how to introduce new evidence into the practice setting;
- discuss various approaches to the management of change;
- consider how to develop an evidenced-based culture in the practice setting.

Introduction

Whilst EBP is generally accepted as a something to aspire to, in reality changes to practices are not easily made. Although nurses report that they are confident of their clinical expertise, it has been shown that frequently practice is not based on best evidence. Grol and Grimshaw (2003) found that between 30 and 40 per cent of patients do not receive care based on sound evidence. The transferring of evidence into practice is often a daunting, difficult and complex activity. Simply informing people of the latest research findings does not mean that new approaches are adopted and it cannot be assumed that developing people's knowledge and skills will result in practice change – just knowing something does not mean people will choose to do it. For instance, most people know that hand washing is central to reducing infections and yet large numbers of health professionals fail to do this appropriately (see, for example, Haas and Larson, 2008). Changing care delivery and individuals' behaviours and approaches takes time and effort. It is important to be thoroughly prepared before trying to instigate changes. There is no single best way of introducing new evidence into practice; as the type of change required will often dictate to the approach to be used. The intention of this chapter is to give you an overview of the issues you need to consider and the tools that may be of use to you.

What does moving from evidence into practice mean?

There are different terms used for putting evidence into practice. Much has been written about **change management,** where various theoretical models outlining the process and mechanism that can be used for making changes to behaviours and practices are described. The advent of EBP has brought with it the term 'implementing evidence-based practices' which considers how evidence – and in particular research – can be applied in the practice setting. 'Knowledge translation', 'knowledge/evidence utilisation' and 'research implementation' are also used to describe the processes involved in applying knowledge/evidence to a practice setting. Just as there is a plethora of terms there is also a range of approaches and it can seem difficult to navigate your way through these. However the central premise for all of these terms and models is the need to ensure that health professionals' clinical practice is effective and based on sound and current evidence.

Why new knowledge is not incorporated into practice

As highlighted above, much of current practice is not based on sound evidence and yet a great deal of time is dedicated to teaching professionals about the need for evidence-based practice and trying to develop the necessary skills to facilitate this approach. Ferguson and Day (2007) investigated newly qualified nurses' experiences of changing practice and found that while individuals were aware of the need to change certain practices in their own working environment, many felt they were not able to do anything about it due to a lack of confidence and experience and also a lack of support from other staff and/or their manager.

Activity

Consider your own area of practice. Identify those factors which would help and those which would act as barriers to making changes in practice.

Timmins et al. (2012) found that a number of issues impacted on nurses' use of research findings in practice. These relate to a lack of time to engage in EBP activities such as finding relevant up-to-date research; limited skills in relation to application of research to practice; and a perceived lack of support from colleagues and managers coupled with an apparent reluctance to adopt new practices by some. The time between evidence being generated and practice being adopted in a setting could be huge. Often practices will be considered safe, having been based on evidence, but frequently this will be out-of-date theory.

Four main reasons for the under-use of research in practice have been put forward by Rycroft-Malone et al. (2004b):

1 Inability to interpret research findings.
2 Lack of organisational support.
3 Research seen as lacking clinical credibility.
4 Nurses prefer a clinical specialist to tell them of the latest developments.

Thompson et al. (2008) argued that nurses preferred to rely on experiential sources of knowledge. (The proposed 'top five' sources of information and the least used can be seen in Table 10.1.) Yadav and Fealy (2012) support the idea that nurses rely on this experiential knowledge and clinical expertise gained through their own and others' experiences. This type of knowledge is valued because it is specific to the context in which nurses work, as well as readily accessible and patient-centred. Research, on the other hand, tends to be seen as less easy to access, and often not specifically relevant to the sorts of issues nurses are faced with. Nurses also appear to prefer others (such as nurse specialists) to provide them with research evidence rather than seek it out themselves.

Table 10.1 Sources of Information most/least used by nurses

Top five information sources	Least used sources of information
1 Individual patients and personal experience	1 Journals
2 In-service mechanisms	2 'Custom and practice'
3 Nurse education	3 The media
4 Discussions with doctors and fellow nurses	
5 Intuition	

It has been proposed that in any change required at team level and above, 15 per cent of people involved will be for it, 15 per cent will be against it, and the rest will just go along with any outcome for a quiet life. Some people will actively sabotage efforts. Often there is what MacGuire (1990) has described as the 'shifting sands syndrome': at each point of the process of change, barriers are identified by participants to prevent anyone taking the next step ('It can't be done because …'). Bridges (2003) argued the most difficult part of making a change is getting people to let go of their usual practices. People prefer what is 'familiar' to them and are therefore often resistant to what they see as a threat to their normal activities and likely to increase their levels of stress. McPhail (1997) refers to this as 'comfort zones' which nurses have developed over time and are reluctant to change unless they become disenchanted with particular established practices. Moving people out of their comfort zone is not an easy task and can be at the heart of whether change is successful or not. Concerns may relate to beliefs (either real or imagined) about what the change will mean for them and come from:

- fear of the unknown;
- uncertainty about the value of the change;
- a lack of knowledge and/or skills;
- a lack of confidence in ability to meet new demands;
- feelings of powerlessness;
- resentment if change is seen as unnecessary.

Greenhalgh et al. (2004) identified five key factors associated with a person's willingness to implement changes to practice (see Box 10.1).

Box 10.1   Factors associated with individual willingness to change

- Psychological factors – a person's characteristics which may predispose them to innovative practice such as tolerance of ambiguity, intellectual ability, motivation, values and learning style.
- Context-specific issues – the motivation to make changes and 'fit' with individual needs is likely to make someone implement changes in practices.
- Meaning – the meaning the change has for an individual is central to whether or not they will choose to make changes to their practice.
- Nature of the decision – it may depend on other things being in place, such as acceptance by others or being told by others to make the change.
- Information needs – the meeting of these appropriately throughout the process of change.

It has also been suggested that if change is forced on people they may move into their 'panic zone' and because of the emotions evoked will not be able to make the changes proposed (NHS Institute for Innovation and Improvement, 2005). However, if people are only moved into a 'discomfort zone' through the use of appropriate implementation strategies and are then supported through the process, they are more likely to change their practices.

Activity

Imagine that you have been told you need to change a particular aspect of your practice. What feelings would this evoke and what would be your most likely response?

Two further obstacles to change are identified by McPhail (1997) – a lack of shared vision and a lack of forward planning. The lack of a shared vision can lead to a 'them' and 'us' situation where it is felt the 'they' want 'us' to change for no good reason. This may also be supported by a feeling that the work required is not appreciated by 'them' and all the hard work is left to 'us'. Unless there are sufficient numbers of people committed to a change, who share the same vision, then any attempt to implement change is likely to fail. If people have the skills associated with, and see benefits to, implementing a new practice they are more likely to be motivated to make a change. Finally, the lack of forward planning is a major barrier to implementing new practices and is discussed in more depth below.

Upton and Brooks (1995) offer a 'change equation' – $f(D,V,S) > R$.

They suggest that successful change will be achieved where:

A combination of the factors

Dissatisfaction with current practices ⎫

Vision for a better future ⎬ IS GREATER THAN   Resistance to the change

Step are planned to achieve goals ⎭

Table 10.2 Elements required to promote change

Element	Features
Involvement	• All individuals affected by the proposed change – service users, professionals and carers • Creating ownership
Motivation	• Valuing and respecting everyone's contribution
Planning	• Considering all aspects of the change and potential issues • Creating a positive environment
Legitimisation	• Owned by all involved
Education	• Development of necessary skills or knowledge
Management	• Appropriate facilitation and guidance
Expectations	• Having a flexible approach, expecting the unexpected and respecting others' experiences • Anticipating conflict and resistance
Nurturance	• Recognising the needs of individuals
Support	• Active listening to concerns • Providing access to resources
Trust	• Open, honest and clear communication of information

As can be seen there are a number of factors that can impact on implementing changes to practice and there is a need to address these before such changes can be made. The characteristics associated with promoting change are summarised in Table 10.2.

Implementing new practices

According to Akerman (1997) there are three types of change:

1   Developmental – the enhancement or further development of current practices.
2   Transitional – moving from current practice to other desired ways of working.
3   Transformational – radical change which significantly alters the structure and processes of an organisation.

Shanley (2007) echoed this model, proposing different 'levels of intensity' in relation to changing practice. Change can occur on a personal, team, organisation, national or even global level.

If you are a student nurse or a newly qualified nurse the thought of making changes to practice beyond a personal level is probably not high on your agenda. In learning to be a nurse, much of your energy must be focused on learning how to do things appropriately. Nevertheless, it is important to remember that what you learn in Year 1 of a pre-registration course may be out-of-date by the time you are in Year 3. So one of the first priorities in implementing evidence-based practices is to ensure your own practice is based on up-to-date evidence. In making a change at your individual level there is still a need to consider patient preferences, identifying whether:

• the change is appropriate to the patients' expressed preferences;
• patients' are aware of their options in terms of care delivery and able to make an informed choice;
• it is ethically and culturally acceptable to the patient;
• it is practicable in the context you practise in;
• you have the knowledge, skills and resources to implement the change.

There is also a need to discuss changes with practice colleagues to ensure that your actions do not cause friction or difficulties within the care team and do not run counter to the care philosophy of your area of practice.

Five 'pearls' are offered by Butz (2007) which can give a starting point for developing EBP and implementing changes into practice at a personal and team level as well as creating an EBP culture:

1   Personal development – making a commitment to accessing databases on a regular basis.
2   Team discussions – timetabling regular meeting with colleagues to discuss ideas, information and to identify areas for change.

3 Culture of enquiry – promoting and developing an enquiry approach in your area of practice.
4 Research relationships – encouraging the development of relationships that may result in research activities.
5 Disseminate evidence – creating systems for sharing information and best practice evidence.

Activity

Consider the five 'pearls' above. Chose two and identify how you could build these into your work life.

The PARIHS (Promoting Action on Research Implementation in Health Services) framework developed by a RCN project group (Rycroft-Malone, 2004) draws together three elements that are thought to be central to the success of making changes to practice:

1 Evidence – its clarity.
2 Context – its quality.
3 Facilitation – type needed.

For change to be successfully brought about it is suggested that the evidence on which changes are to be based needs to be seen as of good quality, valued and viewed as relevant by both the clinical staff and patients/service users. Grol and Grimshaw (2003) noted the characteristics of the evidence can have a major influence on whether that evidence is integrated into practice, and also argued that some evidence will be easier to integrate into practice than others. If evidence reflects widespread concerns in relation to particular practices, or is seen as supporting professional group values, then it is more likely to be adopted. The quality of evidence also impacts on uptake, for example guidelines that are seen as clear, explicit and straightforward are more likely to be implemented.

If you have identified a body of evidence in relation to a particular issue which has implications for your practice then there is a need to evaluate and synthesise this evidence to identify what needs to be done in relation to your specific area of interest (Fineout-Overholt et al., 2010c). If you have critically appraised relevant evidence as identified in Chapter 6 and created a summary sheet of the relevant papers (see Appendix 5) then you will have an indication of what the key aspects of the evidence are and which papers are or are not applicable to practice. You will need to consider the implications of integrating these findings into practice and whether or not this affects just your own practice or has implications for others. As identified, any proposed changes should be discussed with colleagues to ensure these do not cause any problems within your area of practice. Also any significant changes, as discussed later in this chapter, will require careful planning.

The context in which care is delivered is itself seen as constantly changing. Patients come and go, their conditions change or may deteriorate rapidly, and working with other healthcare professionals brings its own complexities. If change is to be made against this sort of background there is a need for individuals to feel valued, for necessary resources to be readily available and for effective teamwork practices to be in place.

If change in practice is to happen then it needs to be facilitated by someone. The type of facilitation and the facilitator her/himself are seen as central to the process, which needs to be enabling and empowering and must include all the involved parties in the decision-making process. Change at a team level and beyond therefore needs to be facilitated by someone who is prepared to take on the role of a **change agent** supported by senior members of staff. Rycroft-Malone's (2002) work suggested this needed to be someone who is part of the team and present in the day-to-day activities, who can see the change as appropriate and can therefore motivate individuals. The characteristics of a good facilitator can be seen in Box 10.2.

Box 10.2   Characteristics associated with a good facilitator

Flexibility	Commitment
Persistence	Presence
Negotiating	Project management
Facilitation	Persuasive
Credibility	Sincerity
Leadership	Clarity of vision
Good communicator	

It is proposed that the knowledge/skills associated with the change agent role are developed slowly, in a step-by-step and often haphazard way (Greenhalgh, 2006). So if you are participating in facilitating changes to practice beyond those within your personal control, you need to start in a small way and develop the skills and approaches over time.

The process of implementing evidence-based practices

There are various models available to guide the process of changing practice (see Table 10.3 for examples). They all have certain aspects in common, including the need for planning, implementation and evaluation strategies to be in place.

Table 10.3 Models for promoting change

Brady and Lewin (2007)	Lewin (1951)	Metz et al. (2007)
1 Plan – involve all affected by the change. Identify outcomes. Pilot proposals. Identify motivators. 2 Implement – establish a realistic time line with built-in evaluation points. 3 Correct – be flexible and address issues as they arise. 4 Communicate – use multiple ways of keeping people informed. 5 Evaluate – identify impact of changes for both professionals and service users.	1 Unfreeze – recognition of need for change. 2 Moving – making the change by altering behaviours or activities. 3 Refreeze – embedding the changes in practice.	1 Exploration – change/ implementation ideas considered. 2 Preparation – resources needed identified and made available. 3 Early implementation – initial adjustments to implement practices made. 4 Full implementation – all staff have appropriate level of competency and change is fully embedded in activities. 5 Sustainability – skills, knowledge and resources are maintained at required level to ensure changes remain in place. 6 Innovation – consideration of adaptations and other changes required.

Table 10.4 PDSA cycle

Stage	
Plan	• What are the objectives? • Who will do what, when, where and how? • How will you evaluate progress/what data will you collect?
Do	• Implement plan • Note any problems/issues that arise throughout the implementation
Study	• Analyse data collected • Compare data with objectives • Identify what you have learnt
Act	• What do you want to achieve next? • How will you know when you have made an appropriate/successful change?

An approach commonly used with NHS service improvement initiatives is the PDSA cycle (Plan, Do, Study, Act). This is based on the work of Deming (1986) and reflects the scientific process of hypothesis (Plan), experiment (Do) and evaluate (Study). See Table 10.4 for an overview of this.

Iles and Sutherland (2001) suggest that it is important that these aspects are not seen as being separate and discrete stages that are undertaken in isolation. It is likely, no matter how thorough the planning, that issues will arise which have not been considered, therefore planning must remain a continuous process. The implementation phase needs to be evaluated at all points to ensure that what is intended to happen, does indeed do so. As issues arise further planning and then implementation will be needed, with an evaluation of the impact of adjustments made. As Schon (1983) describes, there are areas of professional practice where evidence can be easily used to support practice – the high hard ground – however more frequently practice occurs in 'messy' and 'swampy lowlands' where there are challenging problems which will frequently impact on the rigorous application of evidence to practice.

The planning stage usually involves what is known as a diagnostic analysis. As Nickols (2000) suggests, change is a problem-solving activity which usually starts with a diagnosis of the problem, allowing goals to be identified and strategies by which these can be achieved put in place. The 'problem' considered in relation to EBP is the moving from one practice to another, and therefore the diagnostic analysis will involve a consideration of the area or context within which change is to be made. The idea is to identify any barriers, organisational and/or professional issues which must be taken into account before any attempt is made to implement change. This also allows for the identification of the gap between what is currently happening and what the vision for the future is. Highlighting the gap makes planning the implementation easier and also reduces the likelihood of unforeseen problems and barriers to changing practices.

One of the simplest and easiest approaches to consider the issues around making a change is to use a SWOT analysis – Strengths, Weaknesses, Opportunities and Threats. An alternative to SWOT is the 7S model presented in Table 10.5.

Table 10.5   7S model

Element	Features
Staff	• What is needed – number, skill mix, characteristics (attitudes, values, etc.)?

Skills	• What is needed and what are available in relation to:
	  ○ clinical/technical skills?
	  ○ interpersonal skills?
	  ○ managerial skills?
	  ○ research/EBP skills?

Structure	• What are the current features of the organisation? • What is needed? • What is the 'fit' between the two?
Systems	• What is in place and what is needed?
Strategy	• What is the plan? • What are the priorities?
Style (management)	• What is the current style? • Does this fit with what is needed to achieve the planned changes?
Shared beliefs	• What beliefs and values are present? • What is needed to achieve the planned change? • Is there a gap between the two?

Activity

Identify an area of practice that you would like to change and use either a SWOT (a template is provided in Appendix 1) or 7S model to identify the issues you would need to consider.

An alternative to these two models is the 'how, what and why' approach. These question types reflect the various approaches to change that different people take within organisations – namely their 'mindset'. Working through these questions can help to address all the issues that need to be considered and planned for:

- How do I get colleagues to change from X to Y intervention?
- What do I want to achieve, what changes have to be made, what will indicate success?
- Why is X intervention used and why do we need to change to Y?

Activity

Consider the SWOT or 7S analysis you undertook in relation to your chosen area of practice. Does the 'how, what, why' approach provide information you hadn't considered?

Once all the issues that may impact on implementing change and the resources needed have been identified, planning how to make the change is undertaken. There is a need here to set realistic goals, to identify a time line and draw up an implementation strategy. Changing practices takes time, and all those who the change will affect should be involved, with time to ensure there is adequate consultation and planning.

McLean (2011) contends there is also a need to manage the psychological impact of making the transition from one practice to another. As transitions involve 'endings' it is necessary to consider how best to manage these. She suggested a five-step model which acknowledges the psychological impact implicit in moving from one practice to another. Often people experience anxiety and worry about the implications of changes and without a clear vision of why practices are 'ending' may view previous ways of working through 'rose tinted glasses'. There are three phases to transition: 'ending', when 'old' practices are stopping; neutral, where 'old' practices have not completely finished and 'new' practices are not fully embedded; and a beginning phase when the new practice is fully implemented. McLean asserted that a transition facilitator and/or team should be set up to ensure the transition runs smoothly. Table 10.6 outlines the phases of transition and the role of the facilitator/team during each stage.

Table 10.6   Five stage model for managing transitions

Stages	Roles of the transition facilitator/team
Ending phase	
1 Needs assessment	• Assess 'old' system – so a balanced message is given • Highlight what worked – celebrate achievements • Identify what did not work • Define need to stop – gives a clear view of why things must change • Identify training needs • Identify hidden talents
2 Implementation and assessment of interventions	• Identify interventions to support staff through the transition, particularly the 'breaking away' from previous ways of working • Remind people of the problems associated with past approaches • Highlight the benefits of, and reasons for, making the change
Neutral phase	
3 Needs assessment	• Focus and moving forward to ensure momentum maintained • Reinforce why change is needed, identifying positive aspects • Acknowledge stress and anxiety associated with change • Develop interim policies and procedures • Identify and measure short-term goals • Encourage discussion of thoughts and ideas
4 Implementation and assessment of interventions	• Coaching and mentoring staff in new ways of working and building competency • Monitor staff satisfaction in relation to changes • Provide regular feedback and progress reports
Beginning phase	
5 Assessment and assuring sustainability	• Continue to identify why change was needed • Monitor progress • Ensure agreed outcomes are met and sustained

Implementation has its own specific areas for consideration. Metz et al. (2007) suggest that there are three types of implementation:

1   Paper – where policies are in place but no changes to practice actually occur.
2   Fragmented – new structures are put in place but not targeted at the right people: therefore those involved are unable to develop the necessary skills and again practice remains unchanged.
3   Impact implementation – where strategies and structures are appropriate and are designed specifically to ensure practice change.

As can be seen, not all proposed changes occur and there are a number of barriers to successful implementation of changes:

- perception of research/evidence – this has to be seen as legitimate;
- staff factors – lack of experience, knowledge, skills;
- organisational issues – structure, management systems;
- resources – equipment, staff and so on are not available;
- patient/carer perceptions – preference, level of knowledge, availability of information.

In implementing change there is a need to ensure that all these have been taken into consideration and addressed before attempting to make a change. There is also a need to check progress frequently and ensure feedback is given to people at regular intervals so they are aware of progress and any issues that have arisen. If changes to practice are to be sustained and the practices implemented remain in place, there is a further need to ensure that the necessary resources are maintained and people are rewarded for doing a good job.

Once the change has been fully integrated into practice there is a need to formally evaluate the implementation of the practice, identifying whether the change has had an appropriate impact on care, and the lessons learnt and whether further innovations are needed. You must be able to see whether or not you have actually arrived at the point you intended and whether the planned change is an improvement on previous practices. Without evaluation you could end up with the situation where the 'implementation of the change is a success but unfortunately the patient died'. As identified in Chapter 1 evaluation is different to research and audit and has different goals. Evaluation needs to be planned as part of the process of introducing new practices and taking decisions in the planning phase as to what is intended to be evaluated – the effectiveness of the practice, the processes used, the impact of the changes, or all three. It may also be useful to consider sharing the experience of making changes with a wider audience writing up the project for publication or presenting it at a conference. A wider dissemination through publication/conference presentation may help others struggling with similar problems, whilst at the same time adding to the evidence base for nursing practice.

EBP Activity

Consider the diagnosis analysis you undertook earlier in the chapter and create a possible implementation and evaluation strategy that would enable you to change an aspect of your practice. Discuss the feasibility of your plan with a colleague/peer.

Summary

- The transferring of evidence into practice is a complex activity which takes time and effort.
- Comfort zones develop over time and change is unlikely unless nurses are motivated to change established practices.
- A shared vision is needed if change is to be successful and people need to have the skills and to see the benefits of implementing a new practice.
- Change can occur on a personal, team, organisation, national or even global level.
- Strategies and structures need to be designed specifically to ensure practice changes are sustained.

Further reading

Fineout-Overholt, E., Melnyk, B.M., Stillwell, S.B. and Williamson, K.M. (2010) 'Critical appraisal of evidence: part III', *American Journal of Nursing*, 110(11): 43–51. Gives an overview of how to synthesise evidence.

Fineout-Overholt, E., Gallager-Ford, L., Melnyk, B.M. and Stillwell, S.B. (2011) 'Evaluating and disseminating the impact of an evidence-based intervention: show and tell', *American Journal of Nursing*, 111(7): 56–59. Describes the processes for publishing or presenting finding in a clear and accessible way.

Metz, A.J.R., Blasé, K. and Bowie, L. (2007) Implementing evidence-based practices: six drivers of success. Brief Research-to-Results. *Child Trends*, October; www.childtrends. org. Provides a step-by-step approach to moving evidence into practice.

E-resources

National Institute Service Delivery and Organisation Programme: established in 1999 to develop an organisation, management and service delivery evidence base. Their 'Managing Change' web page contains various useful documents. www.sdo.nihr.ac.uk/ managingchange.html

The NHS Institution for Innovation and Improvement: has a series of Improvement Leader guides aimed at providing people with the skills and knowledge to promote service improvement and innovation. www.institute.nhs.uk

11

Reflection, Portfolios and Evidence-Based Practice

Learning Outcomes

By the end of the chapter you will be able to:

- identify the key aspects of lifelong learning;
- apply reflection as an aspect of EBP;
- bring reflective approaches to practice;
- discuss your personal and professional development needs;
- identify key elements of portfolio development.

Introduction

Evidence-based practice is viewed as not only encompassing the use of appropriate research and literature but also embracing lifelong learning as a way to ensuring practice is evidence-based. **Lifelong learning** is seen as essential if practitioners are to be able to meet the ever-changing demands of practice. EBP requires that health professionals' knowledge and skills development keeps pace with the demands of practice and evidence development. There is, therefore, a need to develop the skills associated with lifelong learning. **Reflection** and portfolio development are central to this process, as they can enable you to identify your learning needs, set goals for that learning and evaluate whether these have been met appropriately. As a nurse there is a need to be open to learning and the possibility of change, which requires you to continually assess your knowledge and skills and areas requiring development. This chapter will help you to consider how you can develop the skills of lifelong learning and reflection and ensure your personal and professional development.

Lifelong learning

The idea of lifelong learning came from general education, appearing in litera-ture in the early 1970s. It was adopted by nursing with the development of the Post Registration Education and Practice (PREP) requirements imposed by the then nursing regulatory body the UKCC (1995). The importance of lifelong learning was emphasised as a response to the expanding role of nurses and fast pace of change evident in healthcare settings. The NMC (2002) stated that the principles of lifelong learning were 'increasingly important to all registered prac-titioners' and required all nurses to develop their knowledge and skills, demon-strating this through a portfolio of learning and facilitating it by engaging in clinical supervision.

Claxton (1999) describes lifelong learning as the ability to identify:

- your learning needs;
- the goals and resources needed to achieve them;
- your strengths and weaknesses;
- your blind spots, inherent assumptions and behaviours;
- your mechanisms for monitoring progress and motivating yourself when you get 'stuck'.

He suggested that it requires 'resilience, resourcefulness and reflection'.

There are two main ways of learning: mediated – aided by a 'teacher' – and unmediated – through experience. Kolb (1984) proposed that learning from experi-ence is a cyclic process whereby experiences are analysed through the use of reflec-tion to promote learning and generate new ways of working. The four stages are experience, reflective observation, making sense of the experience and testing new experiences. Boud et al. (1985) suggested that people are often unaware of their learning processes, that reflection made these processes accessible and enabled people to use them more effectively and therefore enhance their lifelong learning.

Leaving learning to 'chance experiences' in relation to EBP is not appropriate and a more structured approach which promotes focused experiential learning through the use of self-direction is needed. Self-directed approaches come from theories of andragogy (how adults learn) and are implicit within lifelong learning. It is suggested that adults are self-directive in their learning, namely that they have a readiness for and a motivation to learn, drawing on past experience as a resource for learning.

Self-directed learning involves developing the ability to identify what you need to know and how to go about learning it. Knowles (1990) identifies four key factors that should be considered when identifying learning needs:

1 Assessment of needs – reflecting on your experiences to identify where you are, where do you want to be and what is in the gap between the two.
2 Identifying learning goals.
3 Planning how to meet those goals.
4 Evaluating the outcomes.

Reflective practice

There are many definitions of reflection, however it can basically be said to be the process by which someone actively considers an experience, critically appraising it in light of experience and knowledge and developing new perspectives to be tested in new situations. Therefore reflective practice can be seen as a three-stage cycle (Jasper, 2003):

1 Experience.
2 Critical appraisal.
3 New perspectives.

Williams (2001) put forward there are three types of reflection:

1 Content – related to the description of an issue asking 'what' questions (e.g. what happened?).
2 Process reflection – related to asking 'how' questions (e.g. how did it happen?).
3 Premise or critical reflection – related to exploring the 'why' of things (e.g. why were certain judgements made?).

Reflection provides a structure through which to consider experiences. It also helps in considering 'normal' situations in a different way rather than passively accepting practices as appropriate. Reflection is not something that is built into some people's ways of thinking and not others'; it can be learnt and developed over time.

Jarvis (1992) suggested that reflective practice requires professionals to look at all practice as a potential learning experience by which they ensure their personal and professional development. Critical reflection takes this process one step further by encouraging the individual to identify the differences between their actual practice and what is desirable. Reflection can be seen as a form of self-consciousness, whereas critical reflection is about continual self-critique. It is not an easy thing to do but if it is done well can provide many benefits. Reflection is seen as helping to:

- bridge the theory/practice gap;
- reduce practices based on custom and practice;
- develop an understanding of your practice, the decisions made, the lessons learnt and the implication of these for future practice;
- ensure that care remains patient-centred and based in the patient experience.

Knowledge occurs in the form of either technical rationality (knowing facts) or professional artistry (intuitive knowledge), and both are needed if you are to practise effectively. These can be brought together through reflective processes (Schon, 1983). Critical reflection can provide the opportunity to learn from an experience – what is known as transformational learning – and to adapt practice rather than endlessly repeating the same activity. There are various models available (see Table 11.1 for examples) and different ways of undertaking reflection (see Table 11.2 for examples). Whilst these all share the same basic element, the best way to approach reflection is to find a way that suits your style of thinking and working.

Table 11.1 Examples of reflective models

Gibbs (1988) reflective cycle	Boud et al. (1985)	John (2006)	Borton (1970)
1 **Description** – what happened	1 Experience	1 **Description** of experience – 'what is significant?'	1 **What?** is the issue/problem/? Asking questions such as what happened, what was I doing?
2 **Feelings** – what you thought and felt	a behaviour	2 **Feelings** – 'own and others'	
3 **Evaluation** – what was good/bad about the experience	b ideas	3 **Goals** – 'what was I trying to achieve?'	
4 **Analysis** – making sense of the events	c feelings	4 **Influencing factors** – 'what influenced the way I felt, thought, responded (social, cultural, organisational, cognitive, professional)?'	2 **So what?** – does this tell/teach/mean? Asking questions such as 'so what more do I need to know, so what was I thinking, feeling, so what could I have done differently?'
5 **Discussion** – what else could have been done	2 Reflection	5 **Theoretical framework** – 'what theory did or should have informed my actions?'	
6 **Action plan** – what to do now	a consider	6 **Ethical aspects** – 'did I act for the best?'	
	b evaluate	7 **Previous experience** – 'how does this link with my previous experiences?'	3 **Now what?** – Asking question such as 'now what do I need to do next time?'
	3 Outcomes	8 **Looking forward** – 'how might I do it differently?'	
	a new perspectives	9 **Framing** – 'what have I learnt?'	
	b changes in behaviour		

Table 11.2 Different styles of reflection

Method	Types
Individual	Reflective frameworks
	Critical incident analysis
Facilitated	Guided reflection
	Peer reflection
Group	Action learning sets
Clinical supervision	Individual
	Pairs
	Group

Schon (1983) suggested that reflection is undertaken in two ways:

1   Reflecting-in-action – whilst undertaking activities, during the experience of practice. The ability to 'think on one's feet' and apply knowledge and past experience to the current situation.
2   Reflecting-on-action – a conscious attempt to reflect after the event.

He also identifies what he calls espoused theory and theory-in-use. Espoused theory is knowledge that is 'said' to underpin practice and is generally accepted as the appropriate body of formal knowledge on which to base that practice. Theory-in-use represents the theories *actually* used when practising – the beliefs, values and thoughts that direct your behaviour. Sometimes the two are very different. For example, if asked about promoting patient dignity a nurse may advocate the need to ensure privacy, to show respect for individual wishes and to communicate appropriately with an individual, but in performing a task related to personal hygiene may ignore specific patient preference in relation to religious requirements and so on. Reflection can help in uncovering these discrepancies between espoused and theories-in-action and so enable you to examine your own biases and personal perspectives.

Activity

Consider a recent practice experience and reflect on you actions. Identify what theory was available to underpin your action and what theory were you actually drawing on. Is there a difference between the two and if so why might this be so?

As identified in Table 11.2 reflection can either be unsupervised or supervised. Unsupervised reflection is easier to organise and can be done to fit in with your own needs and timetables. In many ways it is less threatening as there are no concerns about what someone may think about what you have done. However, it does mean that there is also no one to challenge your assumptions or work through difficult issues. Supervised reflection is more difficult to organise and more challenging, but does provide an opportunity to share your experiences with someone else and draw on their experience and expertise. Duffy (2008) posited 'four Rs' need to be present to ensure facilitated reflection is conducted appropriately:

1   Getting the Right facilitator.
2   Choosing the appropriate Reflective framework.
3   Readiness to take part in the process.
4   Reflecting on the process.

Activity

Consider what characteristics you would associate with the 'right' facilitator and for what reasons.

Peer feedback is suggested as a way of aiding the reflective process. Here a trusted and valued peer is asked to give constructive feedback in relation to a particular activity or experience. In receiving this 'feedback' another dimension to your activities and an alternative view as to what happened are provided. However, for this to be effective it must be structured and also each party must be willing to be open and honest with each other.

Reflection can be undertaken in relation to a range of experiences. Often it will be incidents that are seen as 'significant' – either because something didn't go as well as anticipated or because something unexpected happened – that are most likely to prompt consideration. However, it is also important to reflect on the normal, day-to-day events as these are the ones where practice becomes 'ritualised' and likely to be based on out-of-date evidence.

Reflective writing/journals

Reflection can be done by thinking through things in a structured way; however writing reflectively can add another dimension to the process. There is something about taking thoughts and reproducing them on paper that provides greater clarity and insight into an experience and a deeper learning experience. It supplies a way of ordering your thoughts and freely expressing your feelings and concerns. It also helps to structure your experience and to make links between various ideas and concepts. You can consider issues in a more objective way, returning to the account of your practice at a later date if necessary without having to rely on being able to fully recall all the details. If you reflect regularly – in a reflective diary for instance – it can provide a log of your activities and allow you to consider if there are recurrent issues that need to de considered in more depth.

Reflective writing should be a creative process that allows full expression of thoughts and feelings, enabling you to explore and clarify the issues surrounding your experience. Therefore it is expected that you write in the first person – 'I did ...' so that you 'own' the experience. One of the barriers to reflective writing is that often writing is seen as part of a specific process (education programmes, practice reports, nursing notes) and therefore people learn to write in a way that is required by others (teachers, mentors, managers). However this form of writing is aimed at meeting your needs and you should find a way of doing this that you feel comfortable with. As with all reflection it needs to be structured if it is to aid in your learning and so you need to find a model that will help you to do this. Box 11.1 provides a framework that may be helpful in your writing. Like all other skills you need to practise this regularly to feel confident in doing it; don't worry that you 'might get it wrong', rather concentrate on finding a way that feels 'right' for you. It is useful to identify specific times when you will reflect and if you are able to make it part of your routine this will soon become an essential component of your practice. It may also be useful, when in the practice setting, to have a pocket notebook with you so you can jot down thoughts and issues as they happen so you can reflect on them later.

Box 11.1   Template for reflection

1 Describe a practice experience, writing a concise account of what you did.
2 How did you feel at the time?
3 What knowledge/evidence did you draw on when undertaking the activity?
4 What sources of evidence are you aware of that could support your practice?
5 Is there a need to consider other forms of knowledge/evidence?
6 What are your learning needs?
7 What sources of information/resources could you access to support your learning?
8 How will you meet your learning needs?
9 What does this mean in relation to your future practice?

An alternative to keeping a written diary could be to create an audio or video diary where you record your reflection electronically. However, if you choose this medium then it is still important to structure your reflection in some way so that it enhances and encourages your learning.

Clinical supervision

Clinical supervision first appeared in nursing some 20 years ago, being proposed as a way of helping nurses to cope with the demands of healthcare delivery. It gained momentum as it became seen as a way of facilitating aspects of government initiatives in relation to clinical governance, and encouraging continuing professional development and improvement through a formal process of professional support. It has also been endorsed by the NMC as a way to improve standards of care and is intended to be a career-long undertaking.

McColgan and Rice (2012: 36) defined clinical supervision as 'a process of professional support and learning that enables practitioners to develop knowledge and competence to improve care'. Clinical supervision is undertaken between two or more people, with one person identified as the clinical supervisor, and involves reflection-on-action and the implications of this for future care delivery. Usually the clinical supervisor will have undergone some form of training to prepare for their role. The aim of the supervision is to discuss and explore an aspect of practice or a particular issue in depth in an attempt to understand what has happened and if different approaches are feasible/possible/available. The clinical supervisor challenges the supervisee's ways of thinking and working, whilst at the same time providing a safe and supportive environment. There are various models available, however the most commonly used are:

1 Educative (formative approaches) – aimed at developing a better understanding of individuals' skills, action and the patient experience.
2 Supportive (restorative approaches) – considers emotional responses and the experience of delivering care.
3 Managerial (normative approaches) – explores quality issues and ensures appropriate standards of care.

All the approaches usually involve the agreeing of a contract that stipulates the format, length and timing of meeting, confidentiality and recording of discussions. Many NHS trusts have policies in place identifying their expectation of staff in relation to clinical supervision and the form it will take.

Reflection and EBP

Reflection is central to all aspects of EBP, from identifying that there is an issue of concern to implementing changes to practice. Mantzoukas (2007) stated that reflection enables us to unlock the unconscious knowledge on which we base practice, bringing these into our consciousness and thereby allowing our decision-making process to become clear. It also enables you to link the knowledge gained through experience with more formal types of knowledge and to then identify areas of concern. Reflection, as discussed in Chapter 4, is an implicit part of clinical decision making and central to implementing changes to practice. Table 11.3 provides a reflective framework to enhance consideration of EBP issues adapted from Ochieng's (1999) model of reflection.

Table 11.3 Reflection and management of change model

Stage	Features
Self-observation	• What does the practice involve?
Self-appreciation	• What are my feelings, beliefs, values in relation to the practice?
Self-analysis	• What is the espoused theory to support practice? • What is the theory in action? • Is there a gap between the two?
Self-contemplation	• What is my experience of this practice? • How do I react when performing this activity? • What concepts underpinned my practice?
Self-conceptualisation	• How do the concepts identified above relate to current evidence related to the practice? • Is there a need to change my practice?
Self-management of change	• What needs to be in place to make the change?
Self-implementation	• What strategies will I use to implement a change to practices?

Reflection can lead to constructive action in relation to planning, implementation and evaluation of change (Page and Meerabeau, 2000). However, there needs to be a clear link between reflection and actions – making changes to one's own behaviour will not come about without a clear and proactive action plan and the motivation to put the plan into action.

'Doing reflection'

In reflection there is no 'one size fits all' approach and as identified earlier you need to consider what works well for you. There are, however, a few basic things that you need to put in place to be successful:

- experiment with different approaches until you find one that 'fits';
- commit to giving time to reflection in whatever form you choose – see it as an essential aspect to your practice rather than an 'add on';
- start small and work up to the big issues;
- be open to new ideas and new ways of thinking;
- be willing to challenge your assumptions and practices.

Activity

Consider your own needs in relation to reflection and create an action plan to structure your learning in this area using the above steps to guide you.

Portfolio

Portfolios have been around for a number of years and have been particularly embraced by nurse education. Various definitions are available. McMullan et al. (2003: 289), for example, defined portfolios as 'a collection of evidence, usually in written form, of both the products and processes of learning. It attests to achievements and personal and professional development, by providing critical analysis of its contents'. Alternatively Brown (1992) proposes it is 'a private collection of evidence which demonstrates the continuing acquisition of skills, knowledge, attitudes and activity of the individual'. All definitions have the same themes running through them – that portfolios are a collection of evidence that can provide a picture of your personal and professional development. As McMullen et al. identified they are usually in written form, however electronic portfolios are becoming increasingly popular.

There are four main reasons for producing a portfolio:

1   Learning and development – to demonstrate progress over time.
2   Professional development – to meet statutory requirements to demonstrate you have kept up-to-date (e.g. for the NMC).
3   Assessment – as part of a course to enable an assessment of learning.
4   Presentation – to showcase your achievements, for example at an interview.

Portfolios are seen as a way of actively engaging people in their own learning, providing a vehicle through which to explore the process and provide evidence of learning.

Portfolios also promote self-directed learning and development, requiring you as a learner to take control of and responsibility for your own learning. In turn they provide a framework for reflecting on your personal and professional development. Most nurses will have had experience of keeping a portfolio as part of their formal education – if you are a pre-registration student or a newly qualified nurse you will no doubt have been required to keep one in some shape or form. The advent of the Agenda for Change career structure (DH, 2006) and the identification of the Knowledge Skills Framework both indicated that a portfolio of some kind is needed to demonstrate learning and the meeting of agreed developmental goals for registered nurses. Using this to direct your own learning in relation to EBP can seem a daunting task. However, there are key approaches that can be adopted to direct your activities – a possible framework is proposed below:

1 Reflect on a practice issue to provide a view of where you are and where you want to be and therefore your learning needs.
2 Identify learning goals to be achieved through the use of frameworks such as SMART (Box 11.2).
3 Undertake a SWOT analysis to help you to identify which issues are likely to impact on your ability to meet your goals (see template in Appendix 1); this will enable you to generate an action plan (see template in Appendix 9) to achieve your goals.
4 Implement the action plan, collecting 'evidence' of your learning.
5 Evaluate your progress and adapt your plan as you develop.
6 On meeting your goal(s) the process can begin again.

If the above steps are followed and the documentation is completed it will provide you with a portfolio of your development and learning over time and enable you to both monitor and provide evidence of your progress.

Box 11.2   Setting goals using SMART

In setting goals there is a need to ensure that these are clear and specific. Using the SMART framework will enable you to achieve this:

Specific – clearly written.

Measurable – written in behavioural terms – what will be seen when you have achieved it so you will know when you have got there.

Achievable – something within your reach.

Relevant – to your context and development needs.

Time limited – clearly identify the time period within which you will meet the goal.

So a goal using SMART might look something like:

Identify if there are clinical guidelines in relation to X practice in Y context using EBP search engine A and CINAHL database by (date in two weeks' time).

Personal development planning

Personal development planning is viewed as a structured approach by which individuals can reflect on their current knowledge, skills and achievements, and plan their personal and professional development needs. Mulhall and Le May (2001) propose that to make the transition to EBP there is a need for individual nurses to actively plan their own personal and professional development to ensure that they have and maintain the necessary skills and knowledge associated with their area of practice. This includes thinking about your developmental needs in terms of further study and experience. A template for a personal development plan is provided in Appendix 10 and it may be worth considering what your education and training needs are to ensure you have the skills and knowledge to be an effective practitioner capable of EBP.

EBP Activity

Identify an area of practice and using the above framework and tools create an action plan for developing your learning in this area.

Summary

- Lifelong learning, reflection and portfolio development are central aspects of EBP.
- People are often unaware of their learning processes, reflection makes these processes accessible and enables people to use them more effectively.
- Self-directed learning involves identifying what you need to know and how to go about learning it.
- Reflective practice has three elements – experience, reflection and action – and thus provides a structure through which to consider experiences.
- There are three approaches to clinical supervision – educative, supportive and managerial.
- Portfolios provide a framework through which to structure learning.
- Personal development planning is a structured approach to reflect on current knowledge, skills and achievement, and plan personal and professional development needs.

Further reading

Cassedy, P. (2010) *First Steps to Clinical Supervision: A Guide for Health Professionals.* Maidenhead: Open University Press. A good introduction to clinical supervision.

Jasper, M. (2003) *Beginning Reflective Practice.* Cheltenham: Nelson Thornes. Provides a clear overview of the various aspects of reflection.

Timmins, F. and Duffy, A. (2011) *Writing your Nursing Portfolio: A Step-by-Step Guide.* Maidenhead: Open University Press. Provides a good introduction to portfolios and reflection and their uses.

E-resources

CETL Reusable Learning Objects: this website provides reusable learning objects (RLOs) related to a range of topics. These are multimedia overviews of various topics. The 'study skills' section contains a number of RLOs related to reflection. www.rlo-cetl.ac.uk/index.php

Conclusion to Part 3

The aim of this section was to provide you with the necessary skills, knowledge and tools to enable you to make changes to your practice as appropriate and ensure your practice continues to be evidence-based throughout your career. Hopefully you have now:

- identified ways in which changes can be made to practice and issues you need to consider before making changes;
- considered how best to reflect on your experiences and use that reflection to enhance your practice;
- identified your needs in relation to lifelong learning;
- developed confidence in your ability to use evidence appropriately in the delivery of care.

This part ends with a crossword puzzle, with clues to words relevant to Chapters 10 and 11. The answers can be found on p. 179.

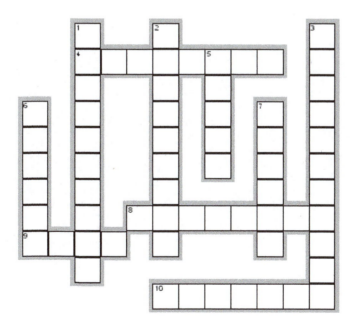

Across

4. theory said to underpin practice? (8)

8. learning aimed at ensuring knowledge/skills are up-to-date? (8)

9. a form of analysis that allows you to identify areas for personal development? (4)

10. zone where people prefer to practise? (7)

Down

1. active appraisal of actions in a structured and critical way? (10)

2. a collection of evidence demonstrating learning and development? (9)

3. someone who facilitates change in practice? (11)

5. framework for defining goals? (5)

6. RCN framework for considering implementation of change? (6)

7. plan identifying how needs are met? (6)

Appendix 1

SWOT Analysis

Strengths *What are my strengths?* *What am I good at?*	**Weaknesses** *What are my current limitations?* *What might I do/think that would stop me meeting my goal?*
Opportunities *What will help in achieving my goal?* *What resources are available to me?*	**Threats** *What barriers are there to me achieving my goal – personal and organisational?*

Appendix 2

Template for Decision Aid

Date prepared ....

Name of intervention	
Aim of decision aid	
Description: *(mode of delivery, frequency, restriction)*	
How does it work?	
Extent of effectiveness	
Goal to be achieved	
What will be required of the patient?	
Benefits	
Risks	
Side effects	
Effect on quality of life	
Sources of further information	
References	
Other options *(it may be necessary to prepare individual sheets for each option)*	

Appendix 3

Forming a Question and Searching for Evidence

Area of interest:..
If your question relates to effectiveness of treatment/care complete the PICO section. If you're considering a topic associated with qualitative research complete the PICo section

PICO	PICo

Population:...................................... Population:...
                                              Phenomenon of
Intervention:.................................. interest:..
Comparison:.................................. Context:..
Outcome(s):..
....
Time:... Time:...
Types of   Types of
studies:.. studies:..
Question:...
....
....

Search Strategy
Free text words:..
....
MeSH/subject headings:...
....
Boolean terms:...
Databases (delete those **not** used):

Cochrane	Joanna Briggs	Trip
NHS Evidence	CINAHL	MEDLINE
PubMed	PsychoINFO	RCN
Centre for Research and Dissemination		Open Grey

Others:...

Summary of information found (summarise each piece of evidence and draw conclusions as to relevance to own practice)

Reflection

Action to be taken

Appendix 4

General Critical Appraisal Tool for Research Studies

Section	Things to consider
Title	• Does it clearly identify the area of study?
Abstract	• Does it contain enough information for you to decide whether or not the paper is of interest to you?
Authors' qualifications	• Are these appropriate for the area of study?
Introduction	• Does it clearly outline the area of interest and give a rationale for the paper? • Is the research question and/or hypothesis clearly identified? • Is a theoretical/conceptual framework identified?
Literature review	• Is there a critical review of the literature related to the area of study? • Is the literature appropriate, up-to-date, mainly from primary sources, and does it include any seminal works associated with the topic?
Conceptual/ theoretical framework	• Are concepts clearly defined? • Is there a fit between the conceptual framework and the research design?
Ethical issues	• Has ethical approval been acquired? • Are the potential risks and benefits discussed? • Are sources of funding and outside interests identified?

(Continued)

(Continued)

Section	Things to consider
Design	• Is the design clearly stated/described allowing for replication? • Is it appropriate to the study? • Are the strengths and limitations debated?
Methodology	• Is this appropriate to the research question/hypothesis and aims of the study? • How are the data to be collected? • What sampling methods are used and are these appropriate to the methodology? • Are issues of reliability, validity, trustworthiness and rigour considered?
Results	• Does it give a clear description of how the results were reached? • Are the results clearly described and presented in a way that promotes understanding?
Discussion	• Are all the results explored and explained? • Is there consistency between the results and the arguments put forward? • Are the arguments logically developed and do they take account of opposing views? • Is the interpretation offered reasonable and does it make sense in light of what you know about the subject area?
Conclusions	• Are these logical and coherent? • Do these 'fit' with the data presented and the arguments presented in the discussion?
Recommendations/ limitations	• Are these presented in a clear way? • Is there a logical link between the findings and the recommendation?
Applicability to practice	• Is the sample used similar to the patients/service users in your area of practice? • Is training required to implement findings? • Are considerations such as costs accounted for? • Do the benefits of changing practice outweigh any identified harmful effects?

Appendix 5

Summary Table of Study Details

Study details (full reference)	Pre-appraised evidence (Yes/No. level 1–6)*	Study design (methodology and method)	Intervention/ phenomenon of interest	Setting (e.g. hosp/ community) geographical location, e.g. UK	Participants/ subjects (number, age, gender, ethnicity, cultural context)	Type of Data Analysis	Key Findings	Quality	Applicability to practice

*Pre-appraised data hierarchy (DiCenso et al., 2009):
1. Systems
2. Summaries
3. Synopses of syntheses
4. Syntheses
5. Synopses of single studies
6. Critically appraised individual studies

Appendix 6

Critical Appraisal Tool for Quantitative Research Studies

Area	Issues for consideration
Hypotheses/ research questions	• Are the research questions and/or hypothesis clear, unambiguous and where appropriate capable of being tested? • Are these consistent with the conceptual framework and research design?
Literature review	• Is there a critical review of the literature related to the area of study? • Is the literature appropriate, up-to-date, mainly from primary sources, and including any seminal works associated with the topic?
Conceptual/ theoretical framework	• Are the concepts clearly defined? • Is there a fit between the conceptual framework and the research design?
Operational definitions	• Are all terms used clearly defined? • Does it identify how variables will be observed and measured?
Design	• Is the design clearly stated/described allowing for replication? • Is it appropriate to the study? • Are issues which may result in bias minimised? • Are the strengths and limitations debated?

(Continued)

(Continued)

Area	Issues for consideration
Data collection methods	• Are these adequately described? • Are the instruments adequately described and appropriate to the study's purpose and design? • Are the instruments used valid, reliable and reproducible?
Sampling method	• Is the population of interest identified? • Are the subject characteristics clearly identified? • Are the inclusion and exclusion criteria clearly identified and appropriate? • Is the sampling approach appropriate to the design? • Is the size of sample identified and adequate? • Are power calculations present where appropriate?
Ethical issues	• Has ethical approval been acquired? • Are the potential risks and benefits discussed? • Are sources of funding and outside interests identified?
Data analysis	• Is it appropriate to the type of data? • Is complete information reported? • Is there adequate description of any subjects who were withdrawn from the study?
Findings	• Are these presented in a clear and understandable way? • Do tables/charts make sense? • Are data described in sufficient detail?
Discussion	• Is it balanced, including all major findings? • Are results considered in light of other research? • Does it address issues of generalisability? • Is there an acknowledgement of limitation?
Validity, reliability, applicability	• Are the results valid and reliable? • Is the relevance for practice identified?

Appendix 7

Critical Appraisal Tool for Qualitative Research Studies

Area	Issues for consideration
Research question and aims	• Is the question clearly stated and appropriate to the topic area? • Are the aims clearly stated and relevant to the research question?
Literature review	• Is there a critical review of the literature related to the area of study? • Is the literature appropriate, up-to-date, mainly from primary sources, and include any seminal works associated with the topic?
Conceptual/ theoretical framework	• Are concepts clearly defined? • Is there a fit between the conceptual framework and the research design?
Design	• Is the design clearly stated/described, allowing for replication? • Is it appropriate to the study? • Are the strengths and limitations debated?
Methodology	• Is a qualitative approach appropriate? • Is a specific approach used and described? • Does the research give a clear justification for the research design?
Reflexivity	• Does the researcher(s) provide a statement identifying their position/perspective?

(Continued)

(Continued)

Area	Issues for consideration
Ethical issues	• Has ethical approval been acquired? • Are the potential risks and benefits discussed? • Are sources of funding and outside interests identified?
Sampling/ participants	• Is the sampling method appropriate and clearly described?
Data collection	• Are the data collection methods appropriate to the research approach and design? • Are the methods described in enough detail for you to understand the process?
Data analysis	• Is the data analysis tool identified and appropriate to the type of data and research design?
Findings	• Are the findings presented in a clear way? • Is there sufficient information to understand how the findings were reached? • Are the findings credible? • Are these discussed in light of other research/literature? • Are the study's limitations identified?
Conclusions	• Are these logical and coherent? • Do these 'fit' with the data presented and the arguments presented in the discussion?
Issues of rigour	• Have steps been taken to ensure the findings have credibility, transferability, dependability, confirmability and authenticity?
Applicability to practice	• Is the sample used similar to the patients/service users in your area of practice? • Is training required to implement findings? • Are considerations such as costs accounted for? • Do the benefits of changing practice outweigh any identified harmful effects?

Appendix 8

Critical Appraisal Tool for Systematic Reviews

Area	Issues for consideration
Question	• Is there a clear and precisely defined question? • Are all terms/concepts clearly and operationally defined? • Are the inclusion and exclusion criteria clearly identified?
Search strategy	• What terms are identified to locate studies, are these appropriate/exhaustive? • What databases were accessed and were these appropriate? • Was a thorough search of all sources of literature undertaken?
Quality appraisal	• How was the quality of the studies assessed? • Is a checklist identified for critical appraisal? • Did two or more people appraise the literature? • Did appraisers provide a rationale for exclusion of any studies?
Data extraction	• Is there evidence that adequate information about sample characteristics was extracted? • Is there sufficient information about findings extracted?
Summarising the evidence	• Where meta-analysis/synthesis is not used is this adequately justified? • Are the methods of 'pooling' data clearly explained? • Is the data analysis thorough and credible?
Meta-analysis	• Are treatment effects reported for all relevant outcomes? • How large is the treatment effect? • Is the heterogeneity of treatment effects adequately addressed?

(Continued)

(Continued)

Area	Issues for consideration
Meta-synthesis	• Were two or more people involved in the data extraction, ensuring the integrity of the data set? • Is a fuller understanding of the phenomenon of interest achieved? • Are the interpretations appropriate and sound? • Are examples of data provided to support interpretations? • Were two or more people involved in the data extraction, ensuring the integrity of the data set?
Conclusions	• Are these coherent and do they flow naturally from the findings? • Is the strength of the evidence discussed?
Recommendations/ limitations	• What recommendations are made? • Are potential limitations identified?
Applicability to practice	• Are implications for practice explored? • How similar is the population of the studies to the patient group you are interested in?

Appendix 9
Action Planning

Goal: *What do I want to achieve?*
Rationale: *Why?*
Action: *How will I go about it?*
Criteria for success: *How will I know when I've got there?*
Evaluation: *What have I achieved and what next?*

Appendix 10

Personal Development Plan

What do I want to achieve? (goals)	How will this help my personal development?	How will I achieve it?	What help do I need?
1. 2. 3.			
Evaluation:			

Solutions to Word Puzzles

Solution to Part 1 Crossword

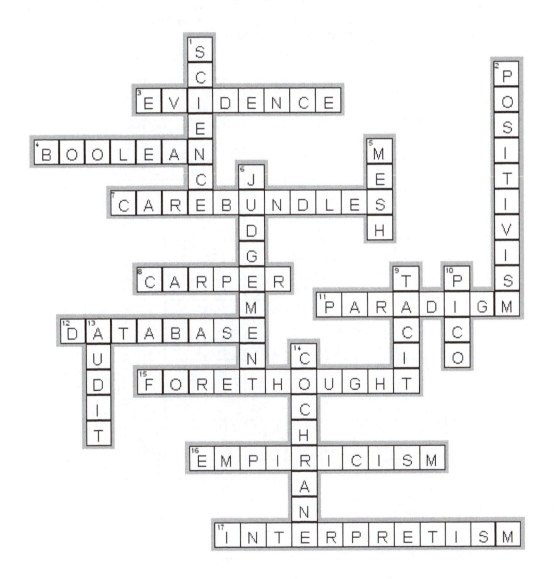

Solution to Part 2 Word Search

Solution to Part 2 Word Search

Hidden words

VALIDITY; RELIABILITY; TRUSTWORTHINESS; CREDIBILITY; DEPENDABILITY; COMFIRMABILITY; TRANSFERABILITY; RIGOUR; VARIABLE; HYPOTHESIS; PROBABILITY; STRATIFIED; ETIC; EMIC; BRACKETING; METAANALYSIS; RANDOMISED; TRIAL; SNOWBALL; MEAN; MODE.

J	T	R	I	A	L	U	O	U	T	Q	T	V	Q	U	X	T	E	V	X
A	G	M	U	Q	V	A	R	I	A	B	L	E	S	E	L	R	O	E	D
S	K	S	Q	Q	L	X	R	I	G	O	U	R	E	B	H	U	M	G	H
K	V	S	J	R	S	J	C	F	D	N	B	T	Y	T	N	S	N	Z	S
K	W	Y	B	F	N	K	O	Q	A	P	F	B	E	R	Z	T	J	R	T
M	A	Z	R	T	O	Q	N	N	Z	R	E	J	U	A	Z	W	D	A	R
O	V	H	A	T	W	E	F	Z	R	O	Z	F	I	N	Y	O	E	N	A
D	S	Y	C	D	B	Y	I	X	E	B	U	F	J	S	H	R	P	D	T
E	M	P	K	W	A	R	R	K	L	A	P	E	Q	F	F	T	E	O	I
R	E	O	E	A	L	E	M	E	I	B	T	T	L	E	F	H	N	M	F
Y	T	T	T	J	L	D	A	F	A	I	K	I	A	R	E	I	D	I	I
A	A	H	I	L	R	V	B	X	B	L	D	C	L	A	W	N	A	S	E
K	A	E	N	D	E	O	I	G	I	I	G	D	N	B	Z	E	B	E	D
E	N	S	G	I	Q	B	L	E	L	T	U	U	L	I	W	S	I	D	S
U	A	I	T	U	R	K	I	E	I	Y	F	G	K	L	Z	S	L	O	S
N	L	S	T	V	P	B	T	Z	T	F	F	Z	U	I	V	E	I	A	B
K	Y	C	W	R	W	J	Y	A	Y	M	E	A	N	T	K	R	T	C	P
L	S	U	J	E	M	I	C	B	A	S	N	K	M	Y	V	W	Y	G	O
S	I	U	F	R	T	Z	Y	P	R	I	V	A	L	I	D	I	T	Y	T
C	S	K	C	R	E	D	I	B	I	L	I	T	Y	T	D	F	R	C	B

Solution to Part 3 Crossword

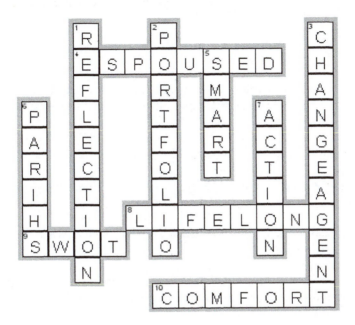

Glossary of Terms

Advanced decisions recording of patient's preferences and care decisions in advance of care needs to ensure these are adhered to if ability or capacity to make decisions is impaired.

A priori knowledge arrived at through reasoning processes.

Authority knowledge coming from a source or person viewed as being authoritative.

Background question generally a broad who, what, where, when, how, why question about an area of clinical interest.

Bracketing a process used in qualitative research, where one's own thoughts and feelings in relation to the study are acknowledged and then 'placed on one side' to allow an unbiased analysis of the data.

Care bundles three or five items of practice evidence grouped together in relation to a particular condition, treatment and/or procedure which have a more positive impact on treatment outcomes than any one single element.

Change agent someone who facilitates change in the practice setting using specific interventions to implement and evaluate evidence-based practices.

Change management the process at promoting change through the use of specific management theories and approaches.

Citation pearl growing a way of identifying literature of interest by using an initial article (pearl) of interest to identify appropriate subject headings.

Clinical audit an approach whereby clinical practices are measured against agreed explicit standards to promote clinical effectiveness.

Clinical effectiveness the delivery of care in the most appropriate and evidence-based way.

Clinical governance the process and structures put in place within healthcare institutions to promote and maintain quality of care.

Confirmability the process of creating an audit trail of decisions taken in relation to analysis of qualitative data.

Correlation studies   quantitative research approach which examines relationships between variables, without manipulation of the independent variable.

Credibility   processes put in place to ensure the findings of qualitative research are seen to be appropriate and representing the participants' experiences.

Critical appraisal   a careful evaluation of the worth, value or quality of evidence.

Cross-sectional studies   research which compares different groups within a population of interest, collecting data at a single identified point in time.

Data saturation   a term used in grounded theory research to indicate the point where no new information is being generated during the collection of data through the use of interviews.

Deductive reasoning   reasoning which moves from general theories to a specific hypothesis.

Dependability   a term used in assessing the quality of qualitative research identifying the need to ensure all participant perspectives are accounted for in the analysis of data and presentation of findings.

Descriptive studies   quantitative research which observes, describes and documents areas of interest as they occur naturally.

Disproportional sampling   a form of sampling used in quantitative research where a larger sample of a particular subgroup (e.g. age, ethnicity) is used than is present within a population. Usually where there is a need to consider the relationship between variables in that group.

Emic perspective   from the individual's rather than an outsider's or researcher's perspective.

Empiricism   a belief that only that which can be observed can be called fact or truth.

Etic perspective   outsider or researcher's perspective, rather than a research participant's perspective.

Evidence   an organised body of knowledge used to support or justify actions and beliefs.

Evidence-based medicine   an approach to the delivery of medical practice aimed at ensuring all activities are based on rigorous evidence.

Foreground question   a focused question formed in relation to a specific issue, looking for particular knowledge.

Gateway site   an electronic device which provides access to specific resources, databases and publications.

Grey literature   literature which has not been formally published, includes theses and/or dissertations, conference proceedings and in-house publications such as leaflets, newsletters and pamphlets.

Hermeneutics   related to meaning and interpretation – how people interpret their experiences within a specific context.

Hypothesis   a simple statement identifying a testable relationship between at least two clearly stated variables.

Inductive reasoning   reasoning which flows from thoughts related to a particular issue to a general theory.

Interpretivism   an alternative to positivism based on the belief that humans are actively involved in constructing their understanding of the world.

Intuitive knowledge   a form of tacit knowledge, which involves arriving at conclusions without being aware of thinking in a rational and logical way to generate that knowledge.

Lifelong learning   self-directed learning in which the aim is to ensure that knowledge and skills remain up-to-date.

Longitudinal studies   research in which data are collected at various points over an extended period of time from an identified individual/group of people.

MeSH terms   medical subject headings commonly used in certain databases to describe the contents of an article.

Meta-analysis   the pooling of data from a number of quantitative research studies to provide a larger data set.

Meta-synthesis   the pooling of findings from a number of qualitative research studies.

Non-propositional knowledge   personal knowledge linked to experience that is used by individuals to help them think and act.

Paradigm   a collection of ideas and concepts providing a theoretical perspective on how knowledge can be generated through research.

Participants   people who make up the sample in qualitative research.

Patient decision aids tools generated through research and evaluation of patients' needs aimed at helping people make informed decisions about their healthcare treatment.

PICO question format used to help to create a search question in relation to a particular clinical issue in which P = population; I = Intervention; C = comparison; O = Outcome.

Positivism a belief that reality is ordered, regular, can be studied objectively and quantified.

Proportional stratified sampling a form of sampling used in quantitative research to ensure subgroups (e.g. by age, ethnicity) within a population are present in a sample in the same proportions.

Propositional knowledge public knowledge, usually given a formal status by its inclusion in educational programmes.

Prospective studies where data are collected in relation to a specific independent variable and the dependent variable is measured at a later date.

Publication bias the tendency to publish studies that report positive results resulting in a reported bias towards the effectiveness of a particular intervention.

Reflection the process by which someone actively considers an experience, critically appraising it in light of experience and knowledge and develops new perspectives to be tested in new situations.

Relevance a consideration as to whether the findings from a study can be applied to the practice setting.

Reliability concerned with identifying if the results of a research study are dependable and replicable.

Retrospective studies research in which data are collected after an event of interest. For example patients' notes may be examined for information in relation to a specific treatment and recovery.

Rich (or thick) description a term used in qualitative research meaning to give a full and thorough account of the research context, the meanings people attach to their experiences, their interpretation of issues and what motivates them to behave/respond in particular ways.

Rigour ensuring that research is of high quality, conducted in an appropriate way, consistent with the underpinning philosophical principles.

Sampling units   people who form the sample within quantitative research, sometimes known as subjects.

Science   a body of knowledge, based on observation, experiment and measurement, organised in a systematic manner.

Search engine   an electronic devise which enables you to search the World Wide Web for information.

Search filter   information put into the database to find the sources of evidence required.

Secondary research   research using data from primary research rather from an original source.

Service evaluation   a systematic approach to gaining insight into patient satisfaction with services.

Shared decision making   a partnership involving the sharing of information between at least two individuals (patient and health professional) to facilitate collaborative decision making.

Subjects   people who form the sample within quantitative research, sometimes known as sampling units.

Systematic review   a rigorous review of research findings in relation to a specific clinical question.

Tacit knowledge   knowledge well known to practitioners but not evident within the research-based literature.

Tenacity   a source of knowledge believed simply because it has always been held as the truth.

Transferability   a term used in qualitative research to describe the tentative application of research findings from one study to another, similar group of participants.

Triangulation   an approach used in qualitative research to increase the rigour of the findings. Entails considering the phenomenon of interest from different angles – usually in terms of its data, methodology, investigators, theoretical framework.

Trustworthiness   whether data from a research study can be considered dependable and credible.

Validity   whether or not the claims made in a research study are accurate.

Variable   is a factor or trait that is likely to vary from one person/situation to another such as weight, temperature, pain, personality traits.

References

Aas, R.W. and Alexanderson, K. (2011) 'Challenging evidence-based decision-making: a hypothetical case study about return to work', *Occupational Therapy International*, 19: 28–44.

Adams, J.R., Drake, J.E. and Wolford, G.L. (2007) 'Shared decision-making preferences of people with severe mental illness', *Brief Reports Psychiatric Services*, 58(9): 1219–1221.

AGREE Next Steps Consortium (2009) *The AGREE II Instrument* [Electronic Version] Available at www.agreetrust.org (Accessed 1 May 2012).

Akerman, L. (1997) 'Development, transition or transformation: the question of change in organisations', in V. Iles and K. Sutherland (eds) *Organisational Change: National Co-ordinating Centre for NHS Service Delivery and Organisations*. London: R & D.

Akobeng, A.K. (2005) 'Understanding systematic reviews and meta-analysis'. Available at www.adc.bmj.com (Accessed August 2008).

Alagiakrishnan, K., Bhanji, R.S. and Kurian, M. (2012) 'Evaluation and management of oropharyngeal dysphagia in different types of dementia: a systematic review', *Archives of Gerontology and Geriatrics*. Available at http://dxdoiorg/10.1016/j.archger.2012.04.011 (Accessed June 2012).

Barker, J. and Rush, B. (2009) 'Rehabilitation and recovery', in M. Mallik, C. Hall and D. Howard (eds) *Nursing Knowledge and Practice* (3rd edn). London: Baillière Tindall/Elsevier.

Barr, O. and Sowney, M. (2007) 'Inclusive nursing care for people with intellectual disabilities using urology services', *International Journal of Urological Nursing*, 1(3): 138–145.

Bartelt, T.C., Ziebert, C., Sawin, K.J., Malin, S., Nugent, M. and Simpson, P. (2011) 'Evidence-based practice: perceptions, skills, and activities of pediatric health care professionals', *Journal of Paediatric Nursing*, 26: 114–121.

Baston, J. (2008) 'Health decisions: a review of children's involvement', *Pediatric Nursing*, 20(3): 24–26.

Bejaimal, S.A., Haynes, R.B., Skariff, S. and Garg, A.X. (2012) 'Finding and evaluating renal evidence: bridging the gap', *Advances in Chronic Kidney Disease*, 19(1): 5–10.

Benner, P. (1984) *From Novice to Expert: Excellence and Power in Clinical Nursing Practice*. Menlo Park: Addison Wesley.

Benner, P., Tanner, C. and Chelsea, C. (1996) *Expertise in Clinical Practice: Caring, Clinical Judgement and Ethics*. New York: Springer

Best, D.E. and Hagen, S. (2010) *Shared Decision Making Interventions for People with Mental Health Conditions. (Review)*. Chichester: The Cochrane Library/John Wiley and Sons.

Billay, D., Myrick, F., Luhanga, F. and Yonge, O. (2007) 'A pragmatic view of intuitive knowledge in nursing practice', *Nursing Forum*, 42(3): 147–155.

BMJ (2007) 'Milestones, tombstones and sex education', *BMJ*, 334 (7585) available at www.bmj.com/content/334/7585/0.2 (Accessed May 2012).

Borton, T. (1970) *Reach, Touch and Teach*. New York: McGraw Hill.

Boud, D., Keogh, R. and Walker, D. (1985) *Reflection: Turning Experience into Learning*. London: Kogan Page.

Bowling, A. (2009) *Research Methods in Health* (3rd edn). Maidenhead: Open University Press.

Braddock, C.H. (2010) 'The emerging importance and relevance of shared decision making to clinical practice', *Medical Decision Making*, 30(5 suppl.): 5S–7S.

Brady, N. and Lewin, L. (2007) 'Evidence-based nursing: bridging the gap between research and practice, *Journal of Pediatric Health Care*, 21(1): 53–56.

Bridges, W. (2003) *Making Transitions: Making the Most of Change*. London: Nicholas Brealey Publishing.

Brown, R.A. (1992) *Portfolio Development and Profiling for Nurses*. Central Health Studies Series No. 3. Lancaster: Quay Publishers.

Buckingham, J., Fisher, B. and Sandue, D. (2008) 'Introduction to EBM'. Available at www.ebm.ualberta.cg (Accessed April 2008).

Bugers, J., Bailey, J., Klazinga, N., van der Bij, A., Grot, R. and Fender, G. (2002) 'Inside guidelines: comparative analysis of recommendations and evidence in diabetes guidelines from 13 countries', *Diabetes Care*, 25(11): 1933–1939.

Butz, A. (2007) 'Evidence-based practice in nursing: bridging the gap between research and practice', *Journal of Pediatric Health Care*, 21: 53–56.

Carper, B. (1978) 'Fundamental patterns of knowing in nursing', *Advances in Nursing Science*, 1: 13–23.

Charnock, D. (1998) *The DISCERN Handbook. Quality Criteria for Consumer Health Information on Treatment Choices*. Abingdon: Radcliffe Medical Press.

Chinn, P.L. and Kramer, M.K. (2004) *Theory and Nursing: Integrated Knowledge Development* (6th edn). St Louis: C.V. Mosby.

Chinn P.L. and Kramer, M.K. (2008) *Integrated Knowledge Development in Nursing* (7th edn). St Louis: C.V. Mosby.

Claxton, G. (1999) *Wise Up: The Challenge of Lifelong Learning*. London: Bloomsbury.

Cochrane, A. (1972) *Effectiveness and Efficiency: Random Reflections on the NHS*. Abingdon: Burgess.

Cochrane Collaboration (2012) *Cochrane Handbook for Systematic Reviews of Interventions*. Available at www.cochrane.org/ (Accessed April 2012).

Cohn, E.G., Jia, H. and Larson, E. (2009) 'Evaluation of statistical approaches in quantitative nursing research', *Clinical Nursing Research*, 18(3): 223–241.

Colaizzi, P.F. (1978) 'Psychological research as the phenomenologists view it', in R. Valle and M. King (eds) *Existential Phenomenological Alternative for Psychology*. Oxford: Oxford University Press.

Collins Dictionary (1998) *Collins Concise Dictionary*. London: Harper Collins.

CONSORT (2012) 'The CONSORT Statement'. Available at www.consort-statement.org (Accessed 30 March 2012).

Cormack, D.F.S. (ed.) (1996) *The Research Process in Nursing* (3rd edn). Oxford: Blackwell.

Coulter, A. and Collins, A. (2011) *Making Shared Decision-Making a Reality: No Decision About Me, Without Me*. London: The Kings Fund.

Coyne, I., O'Mathuna, D.P., Gibson, F., Shields, L. and Sheaf, G. (2011) 'Interventions for Promoting Participation in Shared Decision-Making for Children with Cancer (Protocol)', The Cochrane Library, Issue 2.

Craig, J.V. and Pearson, M. (2007) 'Evidence-based practice in nursing', in J.V. Craig and R.L. Smyth (eds) *The Evidence-Based Practice Manual for Nurses* (2nd edn). Edinburgh: Churchill Livingstone/Elsevier.

Cranston, M. (2002) 'Clinical effectiveness and evidence-based practice', *Nursing Standard*, 16(24): 39–43.

Crib, A. and Entwistle, V. (2011) 'Shared decision making: trade-offs between narrower and broader conceptions', *Health Expectations*, 14: 210–219.

Cullum, N., Ciliska, D., Marks, S. and Haynes, B. (2008) 'An introduction to evidence-based nursing', in N. Cullum, D. Ciliska, S. Marks and B. Haynes (eds) *Evidence-Based Nursing: An Introduction*. Oxford: Blackwell.

Cutts, M. (2009) *The Oxford Guide to Plain English* (3rd edn). Oxford: Oxford University Press.

Dale, A.E. (2005) 'Evidence-based practice: compatibility with nursing', *Nursing Standard*, 19(40): 48–53.

D'Auria, J. (2007) 'Using an evidence-based approach to critical appraisal', *Journal of Pediatric Health Care*, 21(5): 343–346.

Davies, H., Powell, A. and Rushmer, R. (2007) 'Health professionals' views on clinical engagement in quality improvement', The Health Foundation. Available at www.health.org.uk/publications/engaging-clinicians-report/ (Accessed April 2012).

Davies, K. (2011) 'Evidence-based medicine: is the evidence out there for primary care clinicians?', *Health Information and Libraries Journal*, 28: 285–293.

Davis, K., Schoen, C. and Stremikis K. (2010) *Mirror, Mirror on the Wall: How the Performance of the US Healthcare System Compares Internationally*. New York: Commonwealth Fund.

Dawson, D. and Endacott, R. (2011) 'Implementing quality initiatives using bundled approach', *Intensive Critical Care Nursing*, 27: 117–120.

Deegan, P.E. and Drake, R.E. (2006) 'Shared decision making and medication management in the recovery process', *Psychiatric Service*, 57(11): 1636–1639.

Deming, W.E. (1986) *Out of the Crisis*. Cambridge, MA: MIT Centre for Advanced Engineering Study.

Denzin, N.K. (1989) *The Research Act: A Theoretical Introduction to Sociological Methods*. Englewood Cliffs, NJ: Prentice Hall.

Department of Health (1997) *The New NHS: Modern and Dependable*. London: HMSO.

Department of Health (1998) *A First Class Service: Quality in the New NHS*. London: HMSO.

Department of Health (2001a) *The NHS Plan*. London: HMSO.

Department of Health (2001b) *Valuing People: A New Strategy for the 21st Century*. London: HMSO.

Department of Health (2003) *Building on the Best: Choice, Responsiveness and Equity in the NHS*. London: The Stationery Office.

Department of Health (2005a) *Mental Capacity Act*. London: The Stationery Office.

Department of Health (2005b) *Research Governance Framework for Health and Social Care* (2nd edn). London: The Stationery Office.

Department of Health (2006) *Agenda for Change*. London: The Stationery Office.

Department of Health (2007a) *Report of the High Level Group on Clinical Effectiveness*. London: The Stationery Office.

Department of Health (2007b) *Valuing People Now*. London: The Stationery Office.

Department of Health (2008) *Healthcare for All: Report of the Independent Inquiry into Access to Healthcare for People with Learning Disabilities*. London: The Stationery Office.

Department of Health (2010) *Equality and Excellence: Liberating the NHS*. London: The Stationery Office.

Department of Health (2012) *Liberating the NHS: No Decision About Me, Without Me*. London: The Stationery Office.

DiCenso, A., Cullum, N. and Ciliska, D. (2008) 'Implementing evidence-based nursing: some misconceptions', in N. Cullum, D. Ciliska, S. Marks and B. Haynes (eds) *Evidence-Based Nursing: An Introduction*. Oxford: Blackwell Publishing.

DiCenso, A., Bayley, L. and Haynes, R.B. (2009) 'Accessing pre-appraised evidence: fine-tuning the 5S model into a 6S model', *Evidence-Based Nursing*, 12 (4): 99–101.

Dowding, D. and Thompson, C. (2004) 'Using judgement to improve accuracy of decision-making', *Nursing Times*, 100(22): 42–44.

Drake, R.E., Deegan, P.E., Woltmann, E., Haslett, W., Drake, T. and Rapp, C.A. (2012) 'Comprehensive electronic decision support systems', *Psychiatric Services*, 61: 714–717.

Duffy, A. (2008) 'Guided reflection: a discussion of the essential components', *British Journal of Nursing*, 17(5): 334–339.

Eraut, M. (2000) 'Non-formal learning and tacit knowledge in professional work', *British Journal of Educational Psychology*, 70: 113–136.

Ervin, N.E. and Pierangeli, L.T. (2005) 'The concept of decisional control: building the base for evidence-based nursing practice', *Worldviews on Evidence-Based Nursing*, 2(1): 16–24.

Evans, D. and Pearson, A. (2001) 'Systematic reviews of qualitative research', *Clinical Effectiveness in Nursing*, 5: 111–119.

Facione, P.A. (2007) *Critical Thinking, What it is and Why it Counts*. Available at www.gustrength.com/criticalthinking:facione1 (Accessed April 2012).

Ferguson, L.M. and Day, R.A. (2007) 'Challenges for new nurses in evidence-based practice', *Journal of Nurse Management*, 15: 107–113.

Field, N.J. and Lohr, K.N. (1990) *Clinical Practice Guidelines: Directions for a New Programme*. Washington, DC: Institute of Medicine.

Fineout-Overholt, E., Melnyk, B.M., Stillwell, S.B. and Williamson, K.M. (2010a) 'Critical appraisal of evidence: part 1', *American Journal of Nursing*, 110(7): 47–52.

Fineout-Overholt, E., Melnyk, B.M., Stillwell, S.B. and Williamson, K.M. (2010b) 'Critical appraisal of evidence: part 2', *American Journal of Nursing*, 110(9): 41–48.

Fineout-Overholt, E., Melnyk, B.M., Stillwell, S.B. and Williamson, K.M. (2010c) 'Critical appraisal of evidence: part III', *American Journal of Nursing*, 110(11): 43–51.

Finlayson, K. and Dixon, A. (2008) 'Qualitative meta-synthesis: a guide for the novice', *Nurse Researcher*, 15(2): 59–71.

Fitzpatrick, J. (2007) 'Finding the research for evidence-based practice. Part Two – Selecting the evidence', *Nursing Times*, 103(18): 32–33.

Foster, N., Barlas, P., Chesterton, L. and Wong, J. (2001) 'Critical appraisal topics (CATs)', *Physiotherapy*, 87(4): 179–190.

Foucault, M. (1979) *The History of Sexuality*, Vol. 1. London: Penguin.

Franck, L.S., Oulton, K. and Bruce, E. (2012) 'Parental involvement in neonatal pain management: an empirical and conceptual update', *Journal of Nursing Scholarship*, 44(1): 45–54.

French, P. (1999) 'The development of evidence-based nursing', *Journal of Advanced Nursing*, 29(1): 72–78.

Gawande, A. (2003) *Complications: A Surgeon's Notes on an Imperfect Science*. New York: Picador.

Gibbs, G. (1988) *Learning by Doing: A Guide to Teaching and Learning Methods*. London, FEU.

Glaser, B. and Strauss, A. (1967) *The Discovery of Grounded Theory*. Chicago: Aldine.

Glasziou, P. and Haynes, B. (2005) 'The path from research to improved health outcomes', *Evidence-Based Nursing*, 8(2): 36–38.

Grant, G. and Ramcharan, P. (2006) 'User involvement in research', in K. Gerrish and A. Lacey (eds) *The Research Process in Nursing* (5th edn). Oxford: Blackwell.

Greenhalgh, T. (2006) *How to Read a Paper: The Basics of Evidence-Based Medicine* (3rd edn). Oxford: Blackwell.

Greenhalgh, T., Robert, G., MacFarlane, F., Bate, P. and Kyriakidou, O. (2004) 'Diffusion of innovations in service organisations: systematic literature review and recommendations for future research', *Milbank Q*, 82: 581–629.

Griffith, R. and Tengnah, C. (2012) 'Assessing children's competency to consent to treatment', *British Journal of Community Nursing*, 17(2): 87–90.

Grol, R. and Grimshaw, J. (2003) 'From best evidence to best practice: effective implementation of change in patients' care', *The Lancet*, 362: 1225–1230.

Guba, E. and Lincoln, Y. (1994) 'Competing paradigms in qualitative research', in N. Denzin and Y. Lincoln (eds) *Handbook of Qualitative Research*. Thousand Oaks, CA: Sage.

Guyatt, G.H. Oxman, A.D., Schuneman, H.J., Tugwell, P. and Knottnerus, A. (2011) 'GRADE guidelines: A new series of articles in the *Journal of Clinical Epidemiology*', *Journal of Epidemiology*, 64: 380–382.

Haas, J.P. and Larson, E.L. (2008) 'Compliance with hand hygiene guidelines: where are we in 2008?', *American Journal of Nursing*, 108(8): 40–44.

Hack, T.F., Degner, L.F. and Dyck, D.G. (1994) 'Relationship between preferences for decisional control and illness information among women with breast cancer: a quantitative and qualitative analysis', *Social Science and Medicine*, 39(2): 279–289.

Hammond K.R. (2007) *Beyond rationality: The search for Wisdom in a Troubled Time*. New York: Oxford University Press.

Health Foundation (2012) *Magic: Shared Decision Making*. www.health.org.uk. (Accessed: March 2012).

Health Research Authority (2009) 'Defining research'. Available at www.nres.npsa.nhs.uk/applications/guidance/research-guidance/?entryid62=66985 (Accessed March 2012).

Hoffman, K., Dempsey, J., Levett-Jones, T., Noble, D., Hickey, N., Jeong, S., Hunter, S. and Norton, C. (2010) 'The design and implementation of an Interactive Computerised Decision Support Framework (ICDSF) as a strategy to improve nursing students' clinical reasoning skills', *Nurse Education Today*, 31(6): 587–594.

Huntington, A.D. and Gilmour, J.A. (2001) 'Rethinking representations, rewriting nursing texts: possibilities through feminism and Foucauldian thought', *Journal of Advanced Nursing*, 35(6): 902–908.

Iles V. and Sutherland, K. (2001) *Managing Change in the NHS. Organisational Change: A Review for Health Care Managers, Professionals and Researchers*. London: National Co-ordinating Centre for NHS Service Delivery and Organisation. Available at www.sdo.nihr.ac.uk/managingchange.html (Accessed March 2012).

Ingersoll, G.L. (2000) 'Evidence-based nursing: what it is and what it isn't', *Nursing Outlook*, 48: 151–152.

Institute for Healthcare Improvement (2012) 'What is a bundle?' Available at www.ihi.org/knowledge/Pages/ImprovementStories/WhatIsaBundle.aspx (Accessed 7 May 2012).

Jarvis, P. (1992) 'Reflective practice and nursing', *Nurse Education Today*, 12: 174–181.

Jasper, M. (2003) *Beginning Reflective Practice*. Cheltenham: Nelson Thornes.

John, C. (2006) *Engaging Reflection in Practice: A Narrative Approach*. Oxford: Blackwell.

Justice, L.M. (2010) 'When craft and science collide: improving therapeutic practices through evidence-based innovations', *International Journal of Speech-Language Pathology*, 12(2): 79–86.

Kerlinger, F.N. (1973) *Foundations of Behavioural Research* (2nd edn). New York: Holt, Rinehart & Winston.

Khan, K.S., Kunz, R., Kleijnen, A. and Antes, G. (2003) *Systematic Reviews to Support Evidence-Based Medicine*. London: The Royal Society of Medicine Press.

Kitson, A. (2002) 'Recognising relationships: reflections on evidence-based practice', *Nursing Inquiry*, 9(3): 179–186.

Knowles, M. (1990) *The Adult Learner, A Neglected Species*. Houston: Gulf Publishing Company.

Kolb, D. (1984) *Experiential Learning: Experience as the Sources of Learning and Development*. New York: Prentice Hall.

Kuhn, T. (1970) *The Structure of Scientific Revolution* (2nd edn). Chicago: University of Chicago Press.

Lamb, B. and Sevdalis, N. (2011) 'How do nurses make decisions', guest editorial, *International Journal of Nursing Studies*, 48: 281–284.

Lasater, K. (2006) 'Clinical judgement developing: using simulation to create an assessment rubric', *Journal of Nurse Education*, 46(11): 496–503.

Lasater, K. (2011) 'Clinical judgement: The last frontier for evaluation', *Nurse Education in Practice*, 11: 86–92.

Leininger, M.M. (1985) *Qualitative Research Methods in Nursing*. Orlando, FL: Grune and Stratton.

Levett-Jones, T., Hoffman, K., Dempsey, J., Jeoong, S.Y., Noble, D., Norton, C.A., Roche, J. and Hickey, N. (2010) 'The "five rights" of clinical reasoning: an educational model to enhance nursing students' ability to identify and manage clinically "at risk" patients', *Nurse Education Today*, 30: 515–520.

Lewin, K. (1951) *Field Theory in Social Sciences*. New York: Harper Row.

Lincoln, Y. and Guba, E.G. (1985) *Naturalistic Inquiry*. Newbury Park, CA: Sage.

MacGuire, J.M. (1990) 'Putting nursing research findings into practice: research utilization as an aspect of the management of change', *Journal of Advanced Nursing*, 15: 614–620.

Manley, K., Hardy, S., Titchen, A., Garbett, R. and McCormack, B. (2005) *Changing Patients' Worlds Through Nursing Expertise*. London: RCN.

Mantzoukas, S. (2007) 'A review of evidence-based practice, nursing research and reflection: levelling the hierarchy', *Journal of Clinical Nursing*, 17: 214–223.

Mantzoukas, S. (2008) 'The research evidence published in high impact nursing journals between 2000 and 2006: a quantitative content analysis', *International Journal of Nursing Studies*, 46: 479–489.

Mason, T. and Whitehead, E. (2003) *Thinking Nursing*. Maidenhead: Open University Press.

McColgan, K. and Rice, C. (2012) 'An online training resource for clinical supervision', *Nursing Standard*, 26(24): 33–39.

McLean, C. (2011) 'Change and transition: navigating the journey', *British Journal of School Nursing*, 6(3): 141–145.

McMullan, M., Endacott, R., Gray, M.A., Jasper, M., Miller, C.M.L., Scoles, J. and Webb, C. (2003) 'Portfolios and assessment of competency: a review of literature', *Journal of Advanced Nursing*, 41(3): 283–294.

McPhail, G. (1997) 'Management of change: an essential skill for nursing in the 1990s', *Journal of Nursing Management*, 5: 199–205.

McSherry, R., Artley, A. and Holland, J. (2006) 'Research awareness: an important factor for evidence-based practice?', *Worldviews on Evidence-Based Nursing*, 3: 113–117.

Melnyk, B.M. and Fineout-Overholt, E. (2005) *Evidence-Based Practice in Nursing and Healthcare*. Philadelphia: Lippincott Williams and Wilkins.

Mencap (2007) *Death by Indifference*. London: Mencap.

Metz, A.J.R., Blasé, K. and Bowie, L. (2007) 'Implementing evidence-based practices: six drivers of success. Brief research-to-results', *Child Trends*, October. Available at www.childtrends.org (Accessed April 2012).

Michaels, C., McEwen, M.M. and McArthur, D.B. (2008) 'Saying no to professional recommendations: client values, beliefs, and evidence-based practice', *Journal of the American Academy of Nurse Practitioners*, 20: 585–589.

Miller, S.A. and Forrest, J.J. (2001) 'Enhancing your practice decision making: PICO, good questions', *Journal of Evidence-Based Dental Practice*, 1: 136–141.

Moore, L. and Kirk, S. (2010) 'A literature review of children's and young people's participation in decisions relating to health care', *Journal of Clinical Nursing*, 19: 2215–2225.

Mulhall, A. and Le May, A. (2001) *Taking Action: Moving Towards Evidence-Based Practice*. London: The Foundation of Nursing Studies.

Mullhall, P.L. (1993) 'Unknowing: towards another pattern of knowing', *Nursing Outlook*, 41: 125–128.

Nairn, S. (2012) 'A critical realists' approach to knowledge: implications for evidence-based practice in and beyond nursing', *Nursing Inquiry*, 19(1): 6–17.

National Institute for Health and Clinical Excellence (2009) *Schizophrenia: Care Interventions in the Treatment and Management of Schizophrenia in Adults in Primary and Secondary Care* (Updated Edition). Clinical Guideline No. 82. London: NICE.

NHS Executive (1996) *Promoting Clinical Effectiveness. A Framework for Action in and through the NHS*. Leeds: NHS Executive.

NHS Institute for Innovation and Improvement (2005) *Improvement Leaders' Guide. Managing the Human Dimensions of Change. Personal and Organisational Development*. Available at www.institute.nhs.uk/improvementleadersguides.

NHS Public Health Resource Unit (2007) *Critical Appraisal Skills Programme*. www.phru.nhs.uk/Pages/PHD/CASP.hmt. (Accessed March 2012).

Nickols, F. (2000) 'Change management 101: A primer'. Available at: http://home.att.net/~nickols/change.htm (Accessed 2 April 2003).

Nielsen, A., Stragnell, M.S. and Jester, P. (2007) 'Guide for reflection using the Clinical Judgement Model', *Journal of Nursing Education*, 46(11): 513–516.

Nieswiadomy, R.M. (2008) *Foundations of Nursing Research* (5th edn). Cranbury, NJ: Pearson Education.

Nind, M. and Hewitt, D. (2006) *Access to Communication* (2nd edn). London: David Fulton.

Noblit, G. and Hare, R.D. (1988) *Meta-ethnography: Synthesizing Qualitative Studies*. Newbury Park, CA: Sage Publications.

Nursing and Midwifery Council (2002) *Supporting Nurses and Midwives through Lifelong Learning*. London: NMC.

Nursing and Midwifery Council (2008) *Code of Conduct*. London: NMC.

Nursing and Midwifery Council (2010) *Standards for Pre-Registration Nursing Education*. London: NMC.

Ochieng, B.M.N. (1999) 'Use of reflective practice in introducing change on the management of pain in a paediatric setting', *Journal of Nursing Management*, 7: 113–118.

O'Connor, A.M., Llewellyn-Thomas, H.A. and Flood, A.B. (2004) 'Modifying unwarranted variations in health care: shared decision making using patient decision tools', *Health Affairs*, 63: 1–10.

Page, S. and Meerabeau, L. (2000) 'Achieving change through reflective practice: closing the loop', *Nurse Education Today*, 20: 365–372.

Pape, T.M. (2003) 'Evidence-based nursing practice: to infinity and beyond', *The Journal of Continuing Education in Nursing*, 34(4): 154–161.

Parahoo, K. (1997) *Nursing Research: Principle, Process and Issues*. Basingstoke: Palgrave Macmillan.

Parahoo, K. (2006) *Nursing Research: Principles, Process and Issues* (2nd edn). Basingstoke: Palgrave Macmillan.

Parkes, J., Hyde, C., Deeks, J. and Milne, R. (2001) 'Teaching critical appraisal skills in healthcare settings', *Cochrane Database of Systematic Reviews*, Issue 3.

Paterson, B.L., Thorne, S.E., Canam, G. and Jillings, C. (2001) *Meta-study of Qualitative Health Research*. Thousand Oaks, CA: Sage Publications.

Pearson, A. (2005) 'A broader view of evidence', *International Journal of Nursing Practice*, 11(3): 93–94.

Pearson, A., Field, J. and Jordan, Z. (2007) *Evidence-Based Clinical Practice in Nursing and Health Care*. Oxford: Blackwell.

Peile, E. (2004) 'Reflections from medical practice: balancing evidence-based practice with practice-based evidence' in G. Thomas, and R. Pring (eds) *Evidence-Based Practice in Education*. Maidenhead: Open University Press.

Petticrew, M. and Roberts, H. (2003) 'Evidence, hierarchies and typologies: horses for courses', *Journal of Epidemiology and Community Health*, 57: 527–529.

Polit, D.F. and Beck, C.T. (2008) *Nursing Research: Generating and Assessing Evidence for Nursing Practice* (8th edn). Philadelphia: Lippincott Williams and Wilkins.

Polit, D.F. and Hungler, B.P. (1989) *Essentials of Nursing Research: Methods, Appraisal and Utilization* (2nd edn). Philadelphia: JB Lippincott Company.

Pope, C., Mays, N. and Popay, J. (2007) *Synthesizing Qualitative and Quantitative Health Evidence: A Guide to Methods*. Maidenhead: Open University Press.

Porter, S. and O'Halloran, P. (2012) 'The use and limitation of realistic evaluation as a tool for evidence-based practice: a critical realist perspective', *Nursing Inquiry*, 19(1): 18–28.

Portney, L. (2004) 'Evidence-based practice and clinical decision making: it's not just the research course anymore', *Journal of Physical Therapy Education*, 18(3): 46–51.

Royal College of Nursing (1996) *The Royal College of Nursing Clinical Effectiveness Initiative: A Strategic Framework*. London: RCN.

Rycroft-Malone, J. (2002) 'Getting evidence into practice: ingredients for change', *Nursing Standard*, 16(37): 38–43.

Rycroft-Malone, J. (2004) 'The PARIHS Framework – a framework for guiding the implementation of evidence-based practice', *Journal of Nursing Care Quality*, 19(4): 297–304.

Rycroft-Malone, J., Seers, K., Titchen, A., Harvey, G., Kitson, A. and McCormack, B. (2004a) 'What counts as evidence in evidence-based practice?', *Journal of Advanced Nursing*, 47(1): 81–90.

Rycroft-Malone, J., Harvey, G., Seers, K., Kitson, A., McCormack, B. and Titchen, A. (2004b) 'An exploration of the factors that influence the implementation of evidence into practice', *Journal of Clinical Nursing*, 13(8): 913–924.

Rycroft-Malone, J., Fontenla, M., Seers, K. and Bick, D. (2009) 'Protocol-based care: the standardisation of decision-making?', *Journal of Clinical Nursing*, 18: 1490–1500.

Sackett, D.L. (2008) 'The need for EMB'. Collated PowerPoint presentations. Centre for Evidence Based Evidence. Available at www.cebm.net/index.aspx?o=1083.

Sackett, D.L., Rosenberg, W.M.C., Grey, J.A.M., Haynes, R.B. and Richardson, W.S. (1996) 'Evidence based medicine: what it is and what it isn't. It's about integrating individual clinical expertise and the best external evidence', *British Medical Journal*, 312(7023): 71–72.

Sackett, D.L., Straus, S.E., Scott-Richardson, W., Rosenberg.W.M.C., Grey, J.A.M. and Haynes, R.B. (2000) *Evidence-based Medicine: How to Practice and Teach EBM*. London; Churchill Livingston.

Sandelowski, M. and Barroso, J. (2006) *Synthesizing Qualitative Research*. York: Springer.

Sanderlin, B.W. and Abdul Rahhim, N. (2007) 'Evidence-based medicine, part 6. An introduction to critical appraisal of clinical practice guidelines', *Journal of the American Osteopathic Association*, 107(8): 321–324.

Schon, D. (1983) *The Reflective Practitioner: How Professionals Think in Action*. New York: Basic Books.

Schon, D. (1987) *Educating the Reflective Practitioner*: San Francisco: Jossey-Bass.

Scott, K. and McSherry, R. (2008) 'Evidence-based nursing: clarifying the concepts in nursing practice', *Journal of Clinical Nursing*, 18: 1085–1095.

Shanley, C. (2007) 'Management of change for nurses: lessons from the discipline of organizational studies', *Journal of Nursing Management*, 15: 538–546.

Sidani, S., Epstein, D. and Miranda, J. (2006) 'Eliciting patient treatment preference: a strategy to integrate evidence-based and patient centred care', *Worldviews on Evidence-Based Nursing*, 3(3) 116–123.

Sidley, G. (2012) 'Advanced decisions in secondary mental health services', *Nursing Standard*, 26(21): 44–48.

Singh, J.A., Sloan, J.A., Atherton, P.J., Smith, T., Hack, T.F., Huschaka, M.M., Rummans, T.A., Clark, M.M., Diekmann, B. and Degner, L.F. (2010) 'Preferred roles in treatment decision making among patients with cancer: a pooled analysis of studies using the control preferences scale', *American Journal of Managed Care*, 16(9): 688–696.

Speziale, H.J.S. and Carpenter, D.R. (2007) *Qualitative Research in Nursing* (4th edn). Philadelphia: Lippincott Williams and Wilkins.

Standing, M. (2008) 'Clinical judgement and decision-making in nursing: nine modes of practice in a revised cognitive continuum', *Journal of Advanced Nursing*, 62(1): 124–134.

Standing, M. (2011) *Clinical Judgement and Decision Making in Nursing*. Exeter: Learning Matters.

Stevens, K.R. (2004) 'ACE star model of EBP: Knowledge translation'. Academic Centre for Evidence-Based Practice. The University of Texas Health Science Center at San Antonio. Available at www.acestar.uthscsa.edu (Accessed 4 May 2008).

Stott, R. (1999) 'Citation pearl growing'. Available at http://newadonis.creighton.edu/HSL/searching/PearlGrowing.html (Accessed August 2008).

Strauss, A. and Corbin, J.M. (1990) *Basics of Qualitative Research: Grounded Theory, Procedures and Techniques*. Thousand Oaks, CA: Sage.

Stillwell, S.B., Fineout-Overholt, E., Melnyk, B.M. and Williamson, K.M. (2010a) 'Asking the clinical question: a key step in evidence-based practice', *American Journal of Nursing*, 110(3): 58–61.

Stillwell, S.B., Fineout-Overholt, E., Melnyk, B.M. and Williamson, K.M. (2010b) 'Searching for evidence', *American Journal of Nursing*, 110(5): 41–47.

Tanner, C.A. (2006) 'Thinking like a nurse: a research-based model of clinical judgement in nursing', *Journal of Nurse Education*, 45(6): 204–211.

Thomas, G. (2004) 'Introduction: evidence and practice', in G. Thomas and R. Pring (eds) *Evidence-Based Practice in Education*. Maidenhead: Open University Press.

Thompson, C. (2003) 'Clinical experience as evidence in evidence-based practice', *Journal of Advanced Nursing*, 43(3): 230–237.

Thompson, C. and Stapley, S. (2011) 'Do educational interventions improve nurses' clinical decision making and judgement? A systematic review', *International Journal of Nursing Studies*, 48: 881–893.

Thompson, C., Cullum, N. and McCaughan, D. (2004) 'Nurse, information use, and clinical decision making – real world potential for evidence-based decisions in nursing', *Evidence Based Nursing*, 7: 68–72.

Thompson, D.S., Moore, K.N. and Estabrooks, C.A. (2008) 'Increasing research use in nursing: implications for clinical educators and managers', *Evidence Based Nursing*, 11: 35–39.

Timmins, F., McCabe, C. and McSherry, R. (2012) 'Research awareness: managerial challenges for nurses in the Republic of Ireland', *Journal of Nurse Management*, 20: 224–235.

Titchin, A. and Higgs, J. (eds) (2001) *Professional Practice in Health Education and the Creative Arts*. Oxford: Blackwell Science.

UKCC (United Kingdom Central Council for Nursing, Midwifery and Health Visiting) (1995) *PREP and You. Maintaining your Registration*. London: UKCC.

Upton, T. and Brooks, B. (1995) *Managing Change in the NHS*. London: Kogan Page.

White, J. (1995) 'Patterns of knowing: review, critique and update', *Advances in Nursing Science*, 17(4): 73–86.

Williams, J. (2001) 'Using reflection in everyday orthopaedic nursing practice', *Journal of Orthopaedic Nursing*, 10(1): 49–55.

World Medical Association (2004) *Declaration of Helsinki. Ethical Principles for Medical Research Involving Human Subjects*. www.wma.net/en/30publications/b3/index.html.

Yadav, B.L. and Fealy, G.M. (2012) 'Irish psychiatric nurses' self-reported sources of knowledge for practice', *Journal of Psychiatric and Mental Health Nursing*, 19: 40–46.

Zellner, K., Boerst, C.J. and Tabb, W. (2007) 'Statistics used in current nursing research', *Journal of Nurse Education*, 46(2): 55–59.

Index